Before and After Bariatric Surgery

Delicious Recipes for Successful Weight Loss

BY

Christina Tosch

Copyright 2021 Christina Tosch

Copyright Notes

This Book may not be reproduced, in part or in whole, without explicit permission and agreement by the Author by any means. This includes but is not limited to print, electronic media, scanning, photocopying or file sharing.

The Author has made every effort to ensure accuracy of information in the Book but assumes no responsibility should personal or commercial damage arise in the case of misinterpretation or misunderstanding. All suggestions, instructions and guidelines expressed in the Book are meant for informational purposes only, and the Reader assumes any and all risk when following said information.

Table of Contents

Introduction 6

Phase 1: Clear and Full Liquids 8

    Beef Bone Broth 9

    Carrot, Apple, and Ginger Juice 11

    Chai Tea 13

    Green Tea 16

    Homemade Chicken Broth 18

    Lemon Thyme Tea 21

    Minty Lime Infusion 23

    Vanilla and Cinnamon Swirl Protein Popsicles 25

    Watermelon and Lime Popsicles 27

    White Chocolate Protein Shake 29

Phase 2: Pureed Foods 31

    Butternut Squash and Thyme Soup 32

    Cauliflower Puree 35

    Green Pea Soup 37

Italian Chicken Puree 40

Mexican Egg Puree 42

Pureed Chicken Salad.. 44

Shepherd-Style Pie 46

Shrimp Puree 49

Sweet Potato Casserole 51

Tuna Mornay 54

Phase 3: Soft Foods.. 56

Avocado Egg Salad 57

Baked Fish with Almond Chutney 59

Cottage Cheese Bake... 62

Greek-Style Turkey Burgers with Homemade Tzatziki Sauce 64

Instant Pot Turkey Chili 67

Quinoa Muffins 69

Tilapia Stuffed Mushrooms... 72

Tofu Scramble 75

Tuna Zoodle Casserole.. 78

Turkey Bacon, Egg and Cheese Muffins 81

Phase 4: Stabilizing Foods 84

    Baked Marinara Chicken 85

    Beef Stew with Apricots and Saffron 87

    Black Bean Corn Burgers 90

    Cauliflower Crust Turkey and Veg Pizza 93

    Chicken Muffins 96

    Family-Friendly Meatloaf 98

    Halibut in Parchment Paper 101

    Middle Eastern Lamb 104

    Shrimp and Raspberry Salad 107

    Taco Casserole 110

Author's Afterthoughts 113

About the Author 114

Introduction

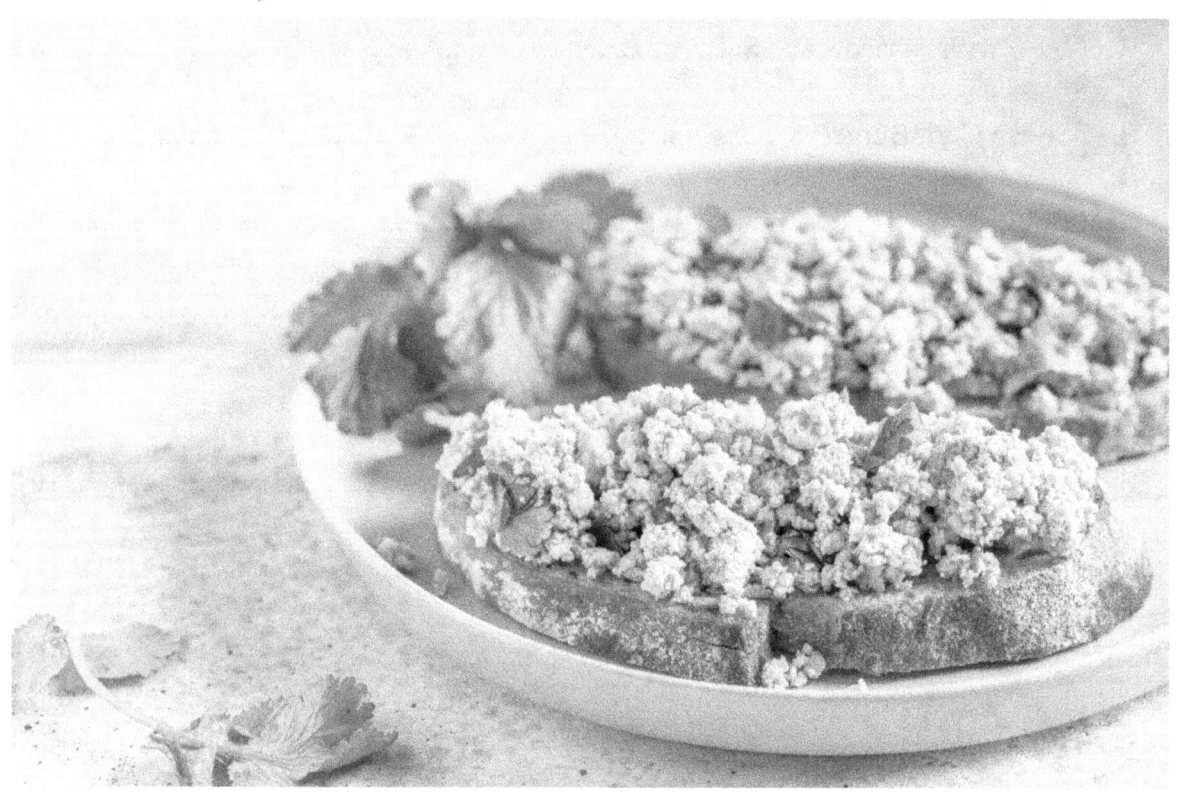

Bariatric surgery is not a magic key to losing weight. It takes a lot of hard work and dedication. What's more, you will have to commit to a significant lifestyle style that includes a specialized diet plan before and after weight loss surgery.

The key to unlocking bariatric surgery weight loss success is healthy eating. From this point on, meals will be small, and this means that every mouthful must count. In which case, the food you choose needs to be well-balanced, flavorful, and nutritious.

So, get those taste buds tingling with these 40 Recipes for Successful Weight Loss that will take you from pre and post-surgery clear and full fluids, pureed, soft, and stabilizing foods.

(About these recipes: Serving sizes on recipes are not necessarily bariatric-sized portions, so check with your dietician for diet plan recommendations, before and after surgery)

Phase 1: Clear and Full Liquids

Beef Bone Broth

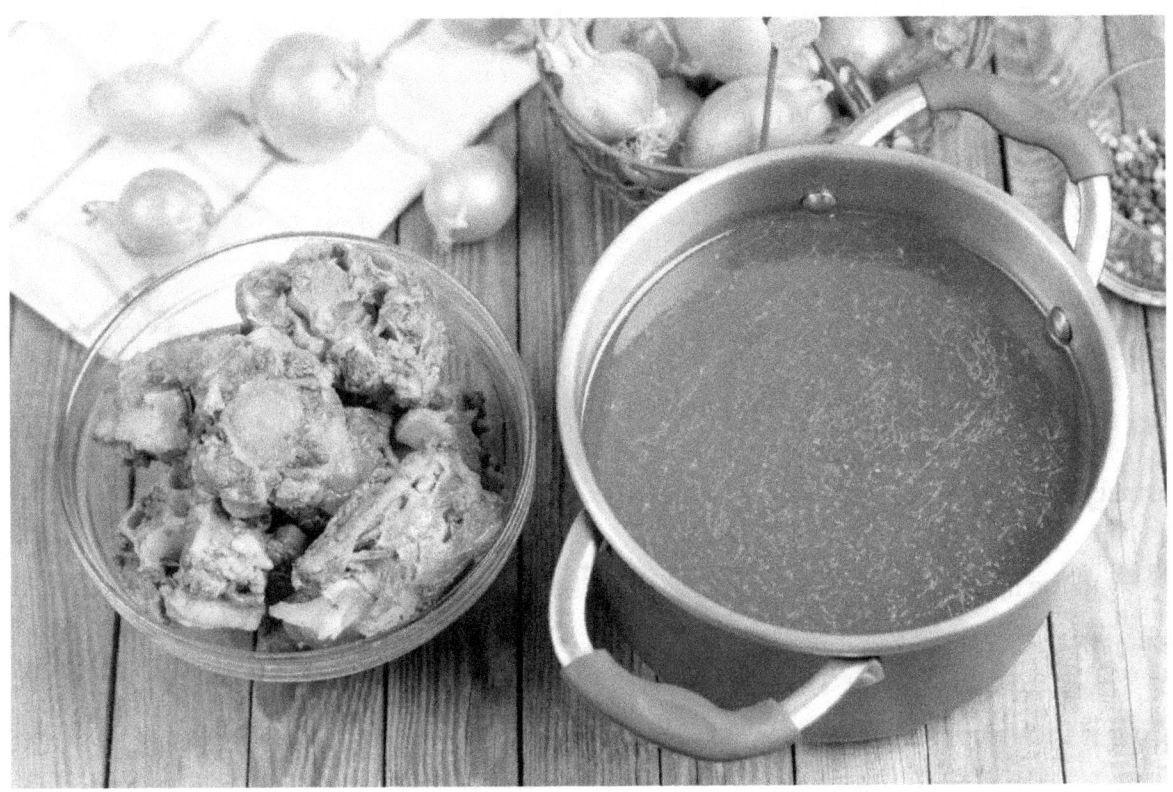

If you are recovering from gastric surgery, this beef bone broth is perfect. What's more, it is ideal before and after gastric bypass or sleeve surgery.

Servings: Approximately 32 ounces

Total Time: 12 hours 10mins

Ingredients:

- 4 whole carrots
- 4 whole garlic cloves (peeled)
- 2 whole stalks celery (trimmed)
- 2 pounds beef bones
- 2 tbsp dried thyme
- 2 tbsp dried oregano
- 2 tbsp dried sweet basil
- ½ tbsp freshly ground black pepper

Directions:

Add all the ingredients (carrots, garlic, celery, beef bones, thyme, oregano, sweet basil, and pepper) to a crockpot.

Pour in sufficient water to cover the ingredients by 1".

Cover, and cook on low for 12 hours.

Strain the soup and enjoy the resulting broth.

Cook's Note: Consult with your surgeon or dietician to make sure this recipe is suitable for your pre or post-bariatric surgery diet plan and or phase.

Carrot, Apple, and Ginger Juice

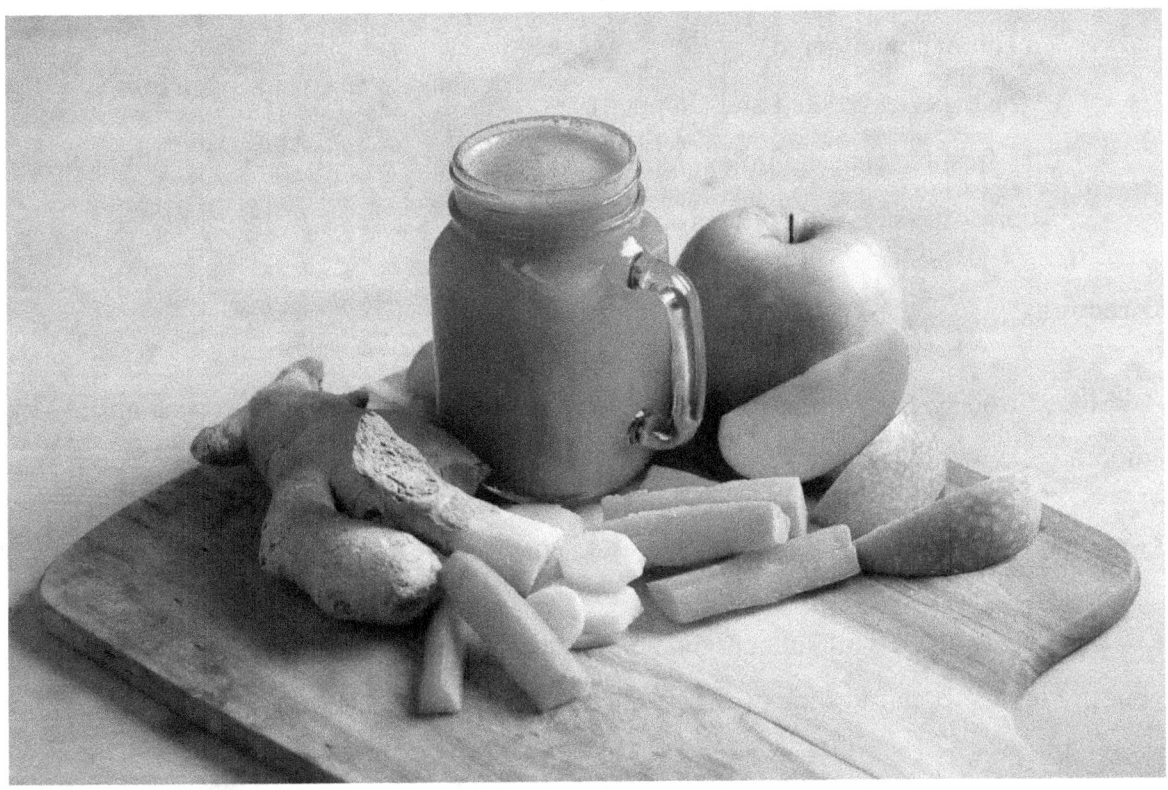

Make those liquids count with this healthy vitamin-packed juice.

Servings: 1

Total Time: 5mins

Ingredients:

- 2 medium carrots (trimmed and peeled)
- 1 medium apple (cored)
- 1" fresh ginger (peeled and chopped)
- 1 tsp freshly squeezed lime juice
- Calorie-free sugar substitute (optional)

Directions:

Add the carrots, apple, ginger, and lime juice to a food blender and process until silky smooth.

Strain the juice through a fine-mesh sieve, sweeten to taste and enjoy.

Cook's Note: Consult with your surgeon or dietician to make sure this recipe is suitable for your pre or post-bariatric surgery diet plan and or phase.

Chai Tea

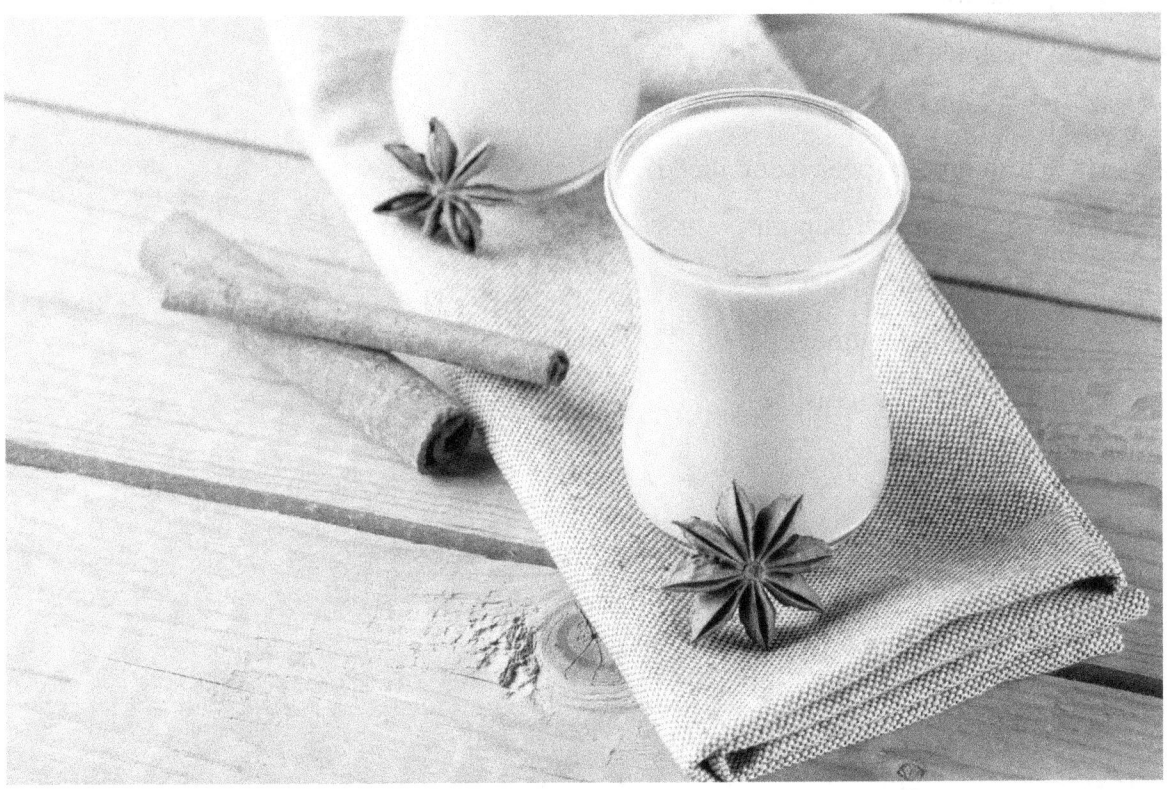

If you are craving a hot drink, this Indian-inspired tea featuring warm spices, non-fat milk, and black tea is the way to go. It's just what the doctor ordered!

Servings: 2

Total Time: 17mins

Ingredients:

- 2 cups water
- 2 black tea bags
- 1 cup non-fat milk
- ½ tbsp ginger (peeled and diced)
- ¼ tsp ground cardamom
- ⅛ tsp ground allspice
- ⅛ tsp ground nutmeg
- 3 whole cloves (crushed)
- 1 cinnamon stick
- 1 star anise
- 1 tbsp vanilla extract

Directions:

In 2 cups of boiling water, steep the black tea.

Over moderate heat, in a pot, bring the milk, ginger, cardamom, allspice, nutmeg, cloves, cinnamon stick, star anise, and vanilla extract to a just boil. You will need to stir to prevent the milk from scorching occasionally.

Add the black tea to the milk-vanilla mixture.

Cover and over very low heat, simmer for 12-15 minutes,

Strain and discard the solids.

Enjoy the tea warm on serve over ice.

Cook's Note: Consult with your surgeon or dietician to make sure this recipe is suitable for your pre or post-bariatric surgery diet plan and or phase.

Green Tea

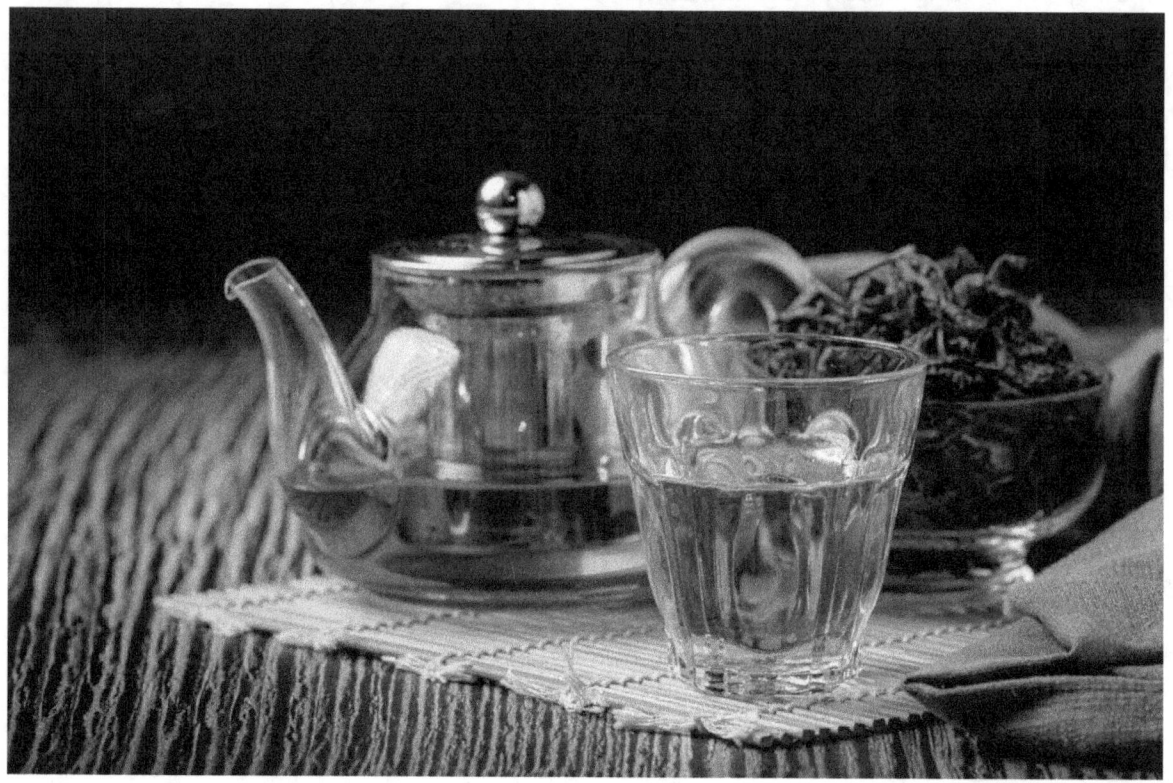

Green tea is ideal for pre and post-surgery and will help you reach your fluid goal of around 48-64 ounces of liquid per day. It is packed full of health benefits and can help you lose weight and reduce the risk of heart disease and diabetes.

Servings: 16 Ounces

Total Time: 5mins

Ingredients:

- 16 ounces water
- 4 decaffeinated green tea bags

Directions:

In a pan, on the stovetop, heat the water to boiling point.

Turn the heat off, add the green tea bags, and steep for 3-5 minutes while covered.

Remove the tea bags and allow the tea to cool.

Sip in 1-ounce amounts and enjoy throughout the day.

Cook's Note: Consult with your surgeon or dietician to make sure this recipe is suitable for your pre or post-bariatric surgery diet plan and or phase.

Homemade Chicken Broth

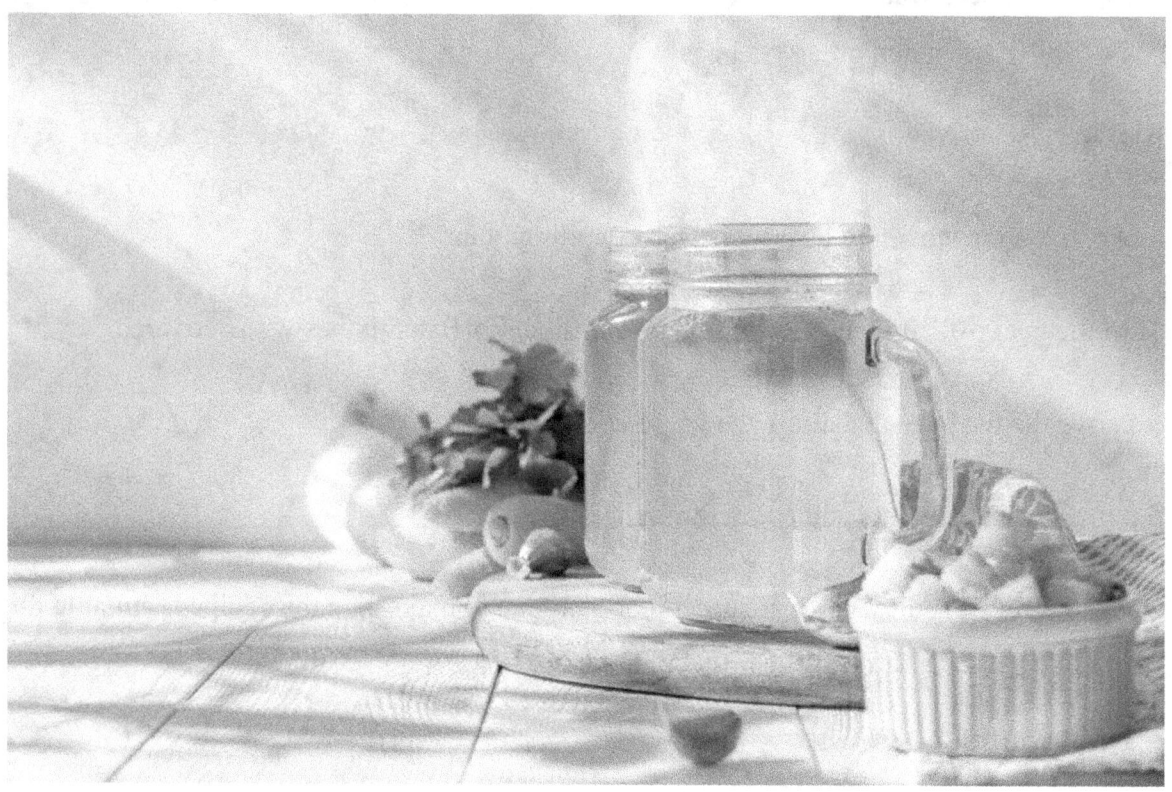

This homemade broth is delicious and nutritious. Better yet, it's a healthy option for anyone following a liquid diet.

Servings: Approximately 64 ounces

Total Time: 8hours 35mins

Ingredients:

- 2 pounds bone-in, skin-on chicken
- 2 large carrots (trimmed and thickly sliced)
- 2 medium onions (peeled and quartered)
- 3 sticks celery (with leaves, cut into chunks)
- 8 whole peppercorns
- 1 tsp dried rosemary
- 1 tsp dried thyme
- 2 quarts water
- Salt (to season)

Directions:

In a pot, combine the chicken with the carrots, onion, celery, whole peppercorns, dried rosemary, dried thyme, and water, and bring to a boil.

Skim off any surface foam or scum, and reduce the heat. Simmer for approximately 2 hours until the chicken can be easily removed from the bone.

Strain the veggies, chicken bone, meat, and herbs from the broth, and remove and discard any solids.

Season the chicken broth to taste with salt.

Allow the broth to cool overnight.

Before serving, skim off any surface fat.

Leftovers can be stored in the fridge or freezer.

Cook's Note: Consult with your surgeon or dietician to make sure this recipe is suitable for your pre or post-bariatric surgery diet plan and or phase.

Lemon Thyme Tea

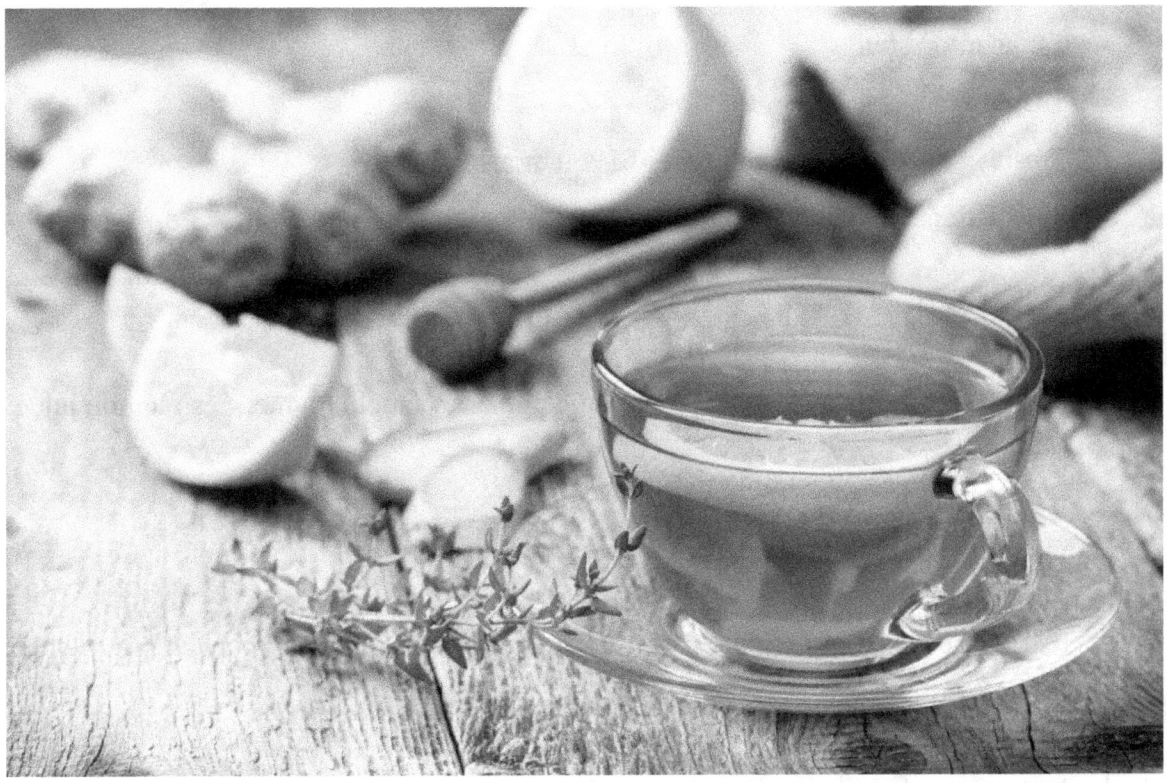

It is essential to stay hydrated, which means sipping fluids throughout the day, and this sugar-free black tea is ideal for anyone following a bariatric diet.

Servings: 32 ounces

Total Time: 18mins

Ingredients:

- 4 cups water
- 1 cinnamon stick
- 1 tsp thyme
- Freshly squeezed juice and zest of 1½ lemons
- 2 decaffeinated black tea bags

Directions:

In a pan on the stovetop, boil the water with the cinnamon stick, thyme, fresh lemon juice, and lemon zest.

Add the black tea bags to the pan, cover, and allow to steep for 12-15 minutes.

Remove the tea bags from the pan, strain through a fine-mesh sieve, pour into a pitcher, allow the tea to cool, and enjoy.

Cook's Note: Consult with your surgeon or dietician to make sure this recipe is suitable for your pre or post-bariatric surgery diet plan and or phase.

Minty Lime Infusion

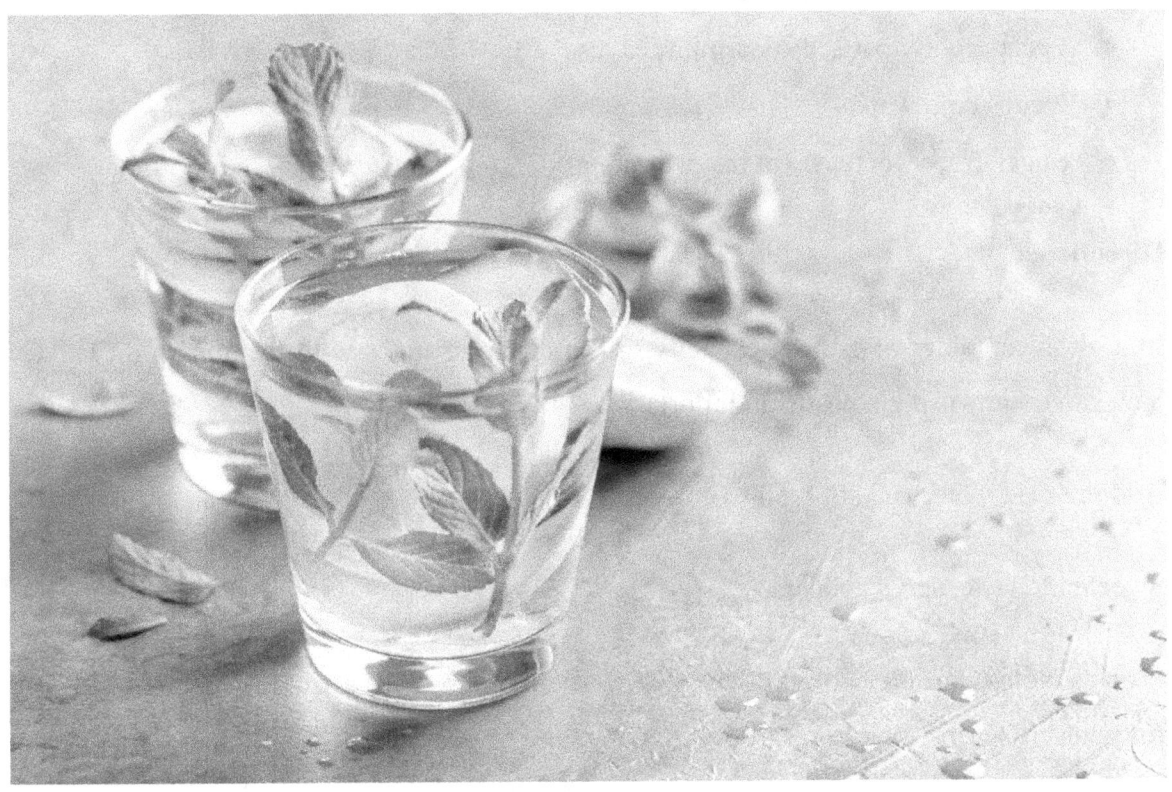

Cool off with this spearmint and lime infusion. It's the ideal refresher and alternative to alcoholic drinks.

Servings: 2

Total Time: 3mins

Ingredients:

- 1 fresh lime (sliced and seeded)
- ½ cup lightly packed spearmint leaves
- 2 cups cold water
- Sugar-free sweetener (to taste, optional)

Directions:

In a glass container of 1-quart capacity, mash the lime slices with the spearmint leaves. You can do this using a pestle and mortar.

Add the cold water and stir well to combine.

Sweeten to taste, serve and sip.

Cook's Note: Consult with your surgeon or dietician to make sure this recipe is suitable for your pre or post-bariatric surgery diet plan and or phase.

Vanilla and Cinnamon Swirl Protein Popsicles

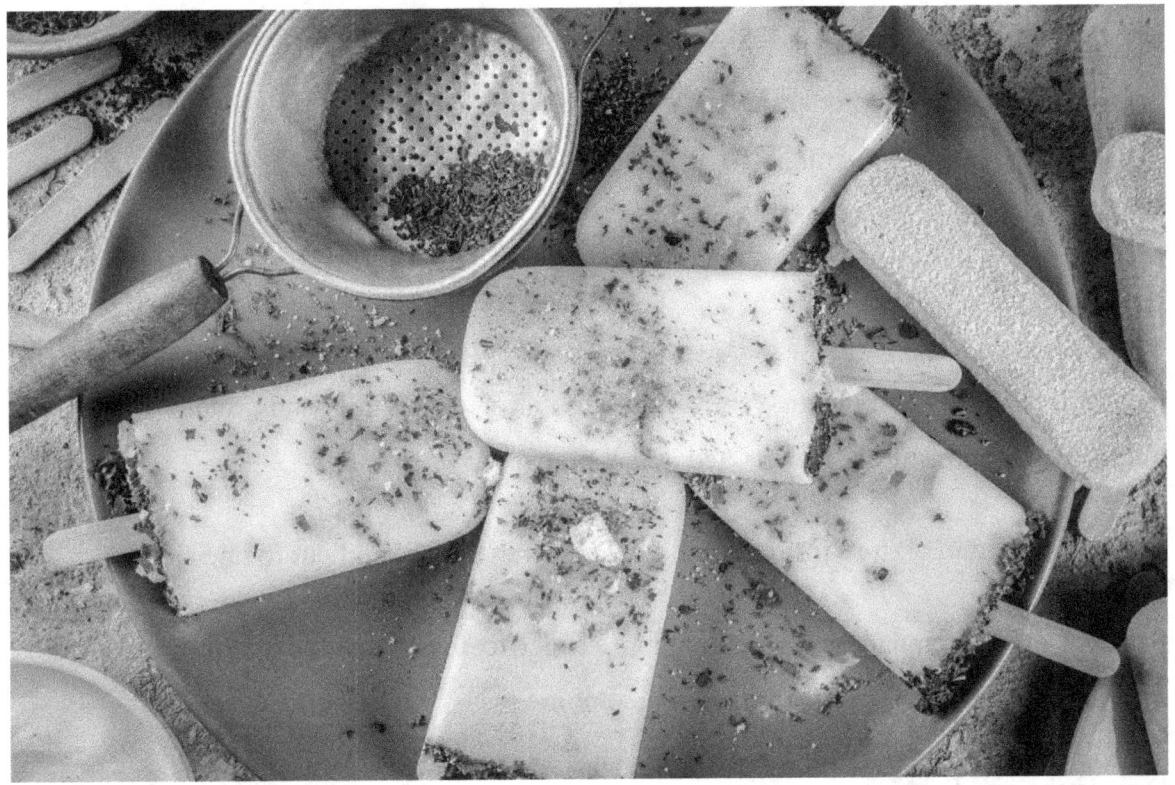

These delicious protein-rich popsicles will help get you well on the way to recovery during the first few weeks of bariatric surgery.

Servings: 4

Total Time: 8hours 10mins

Ingredients:

- 1 ounce sugar-free vanilla pudding mix
- 2 cups unsweetened soy milk
- 2 scoops unflavored protein powder
- 1 tsp ground cinnamon
- 1 tsp cinnamon extract

Directions:

In a food blender, combine the vanilla pudding mix with soy milk and protein powder. On high-speed process until incorporated and creamy.

Transfer ⅔ of the mixture from the food blender into a bowl and put to one side.

Add the ground cinnamon and cinnamon extract to the remaining mixture in the food blender, and on high speed, process until combined.

Drizzle the vanilla-cinnamon mixture over the surface of the vanilla mixture set aside in Step 2, and with a knife, swirl.

Pour the mixture into popsicle molds, and place in the freezer overnight.

Cook's Note: Consult with your surgeon or dietician to make sure this recipe is suitable for your pre or post-bariatric surgery diet plan and or phase.

Watermelon and Lime Popsicles

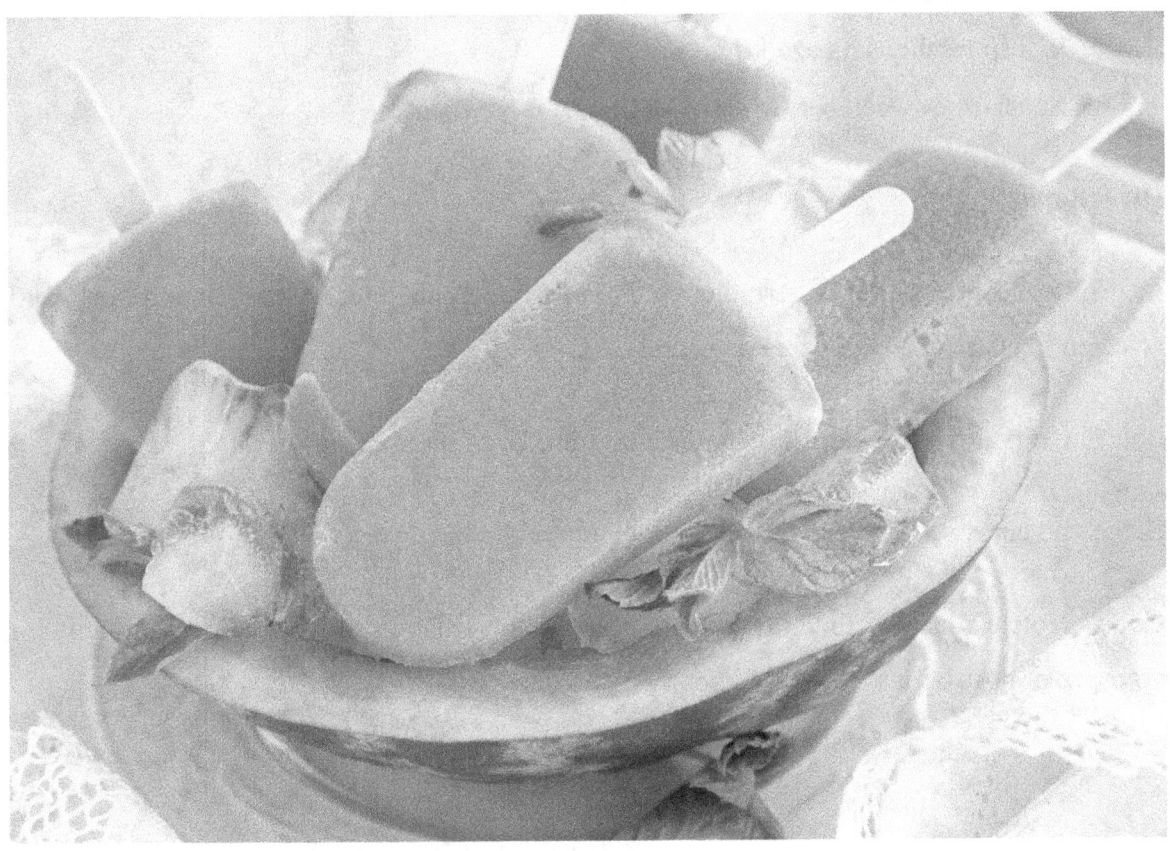

Sugar-free popsicles are a real lifesaver during the early days of gastric bypass or sleeve surgery. Allow them to melt slowly in your mouth before swallowing.

Servings: 4

Total Time: 8hours 10mins

Ingredients:

- 2 cups sugar-free watermelon juice
- ½ tbsp freshly squeezed lime juice
- Sugar-free sweetener (to taste, optional)

Directions:

In a bowl, combine the watermelon juice with the lime juice. Stir to incorporate and sweeten to taste with sugar-free sweetener.

Pour the mixture into 4 popsicle molds, and transfer to the freezer overnight.

Serve and enjoy.

Cook's Note: Consult with your surgeon or dietician to make sure this recipe is suitable for your pre or post-bariatric surgery diet plan and or phase.

White Chocolate Protein Shake

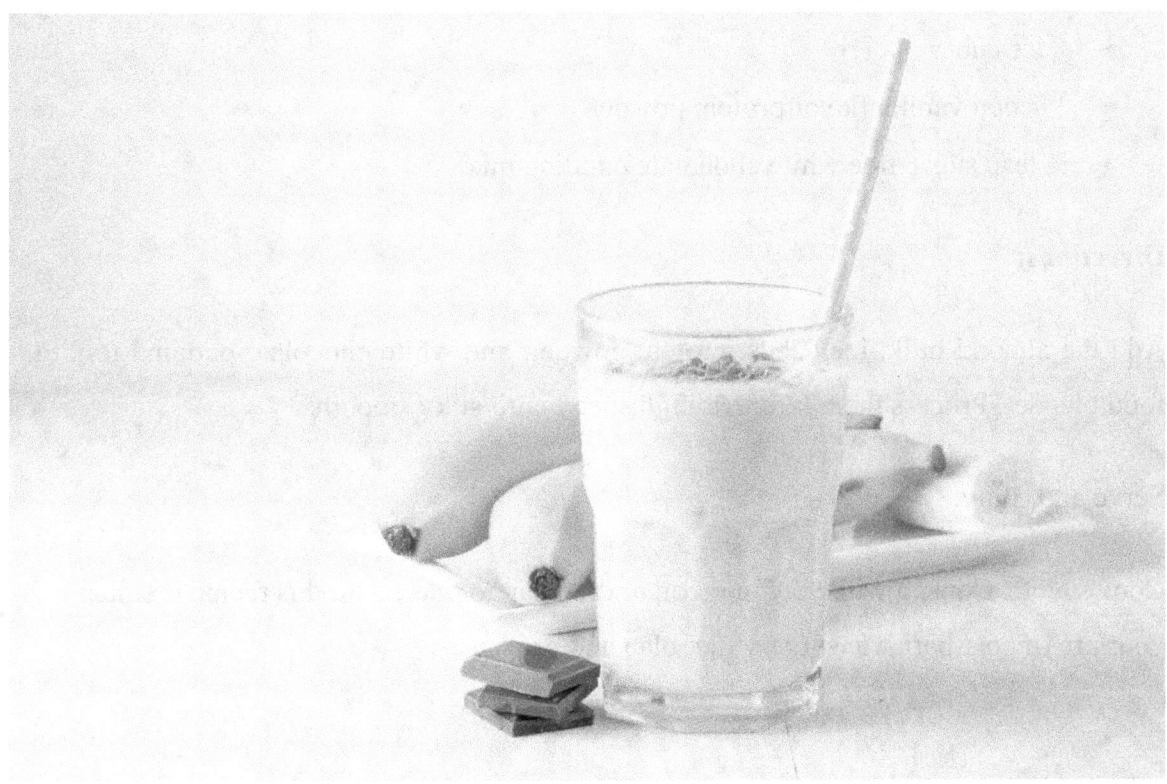

This indulgent white chocolate shake will become your go-to favorite post-op drink. Better yet, protein powders and shakes can help to minimize loss of lean muscle mass and help promote wound healing. Don't forget, though, to sip slowly, and never use a straw!

Servings: 1

Total Time: 5mins

Ingredients:

- 8 ounces unsweetened almond milk
- 6 ice cubes
- 1 scoop vanilla flavor protein powder
- ½ tbsp sugar-free white chocolate pudding mix

Directions:

Add the almond milk, ice cubes, protein powder, and white chocolate pudding mix to a food blender. Process the mixture at high speed until silky smooth.

Serve and enjoy.

Cook's Note: Consult with your surgeon or dietician to make sure this recipe is suitable for your pre or post-bariatric surgery diet plan and or phase.

Phase 2: Pureed Foods

Butternut Squash and Thyme Soup

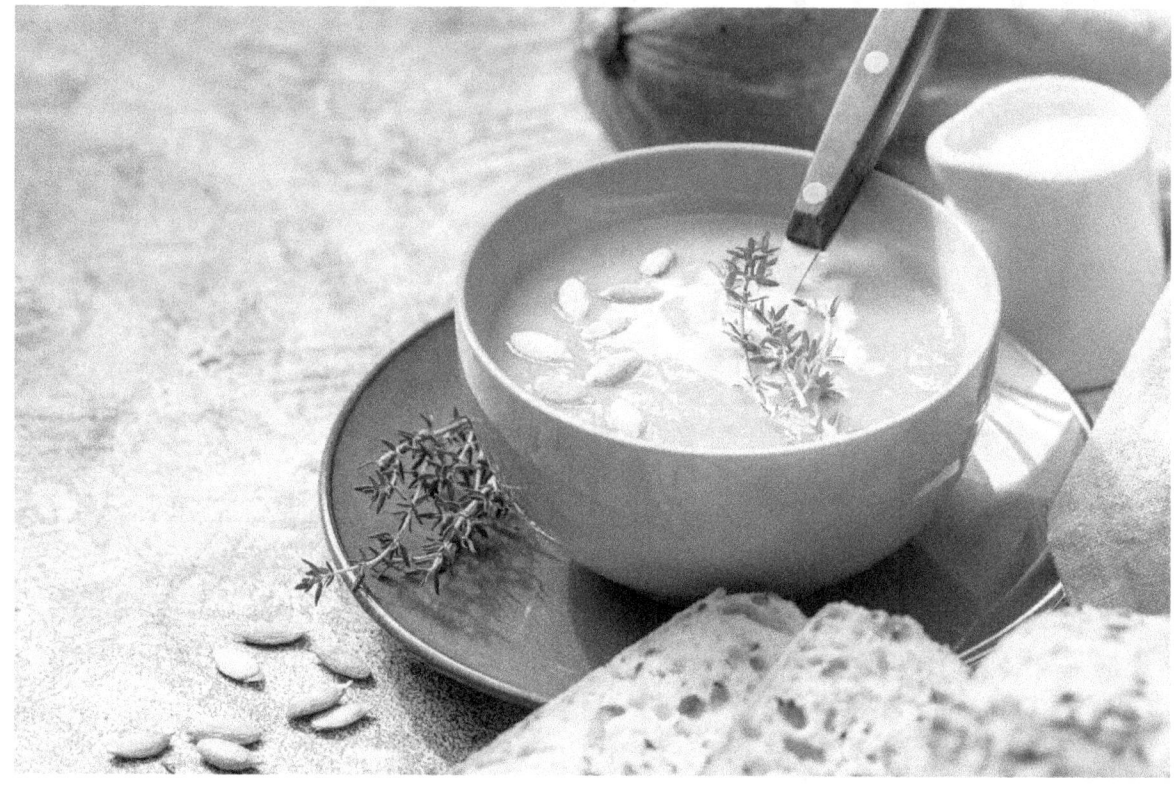

A pureed soup made using lots of fresh veggies is a healthy post-operative meal to share.

Servings: 4

Total Time: 40mins

Ingredients:

- 1 tbsp extra-virgin olive oil
- ½ yellow onion (peeled and diced)
- 2 cloves of garlic (peeled)
- 3-4 sprigs fresh thyme
- 1 butternut squash (peeled, seeded, and cut into 1" cubes)
- 4 cups vegetable stock
- ¼ tsp cumin
- ¼ tsp ground cinnamon
- ¼ tsp nutmeg
- Salt and black pepper

Directions:

In a pan, heat the olive oil and cook the onion with the garlic and thyme for approximately 5-6 minutes, until softened. Add the squash to the pan and sauté for an additional 60 seconds.

Pour in the stock and bring to a simmer, cooking until the squash is fork-tender, for around 25-30 minutes. Season with cumin, cinnamon, nutmeg, salt, and black pepper, and stir to combine. Allow to simmer for another 2-3 minutes. Remove the pan from the heat.

With a hand blender, puree the soup until smooth and creamy.

Return the soup to the pan and allow to warm through.

Serve and enjoy.

Cook's Note: Consult with your surgeon or dietician to make sure this recipe is suitable for your pre or post-bariatric surgery diet plan and or phase.

Cauliflower Puree

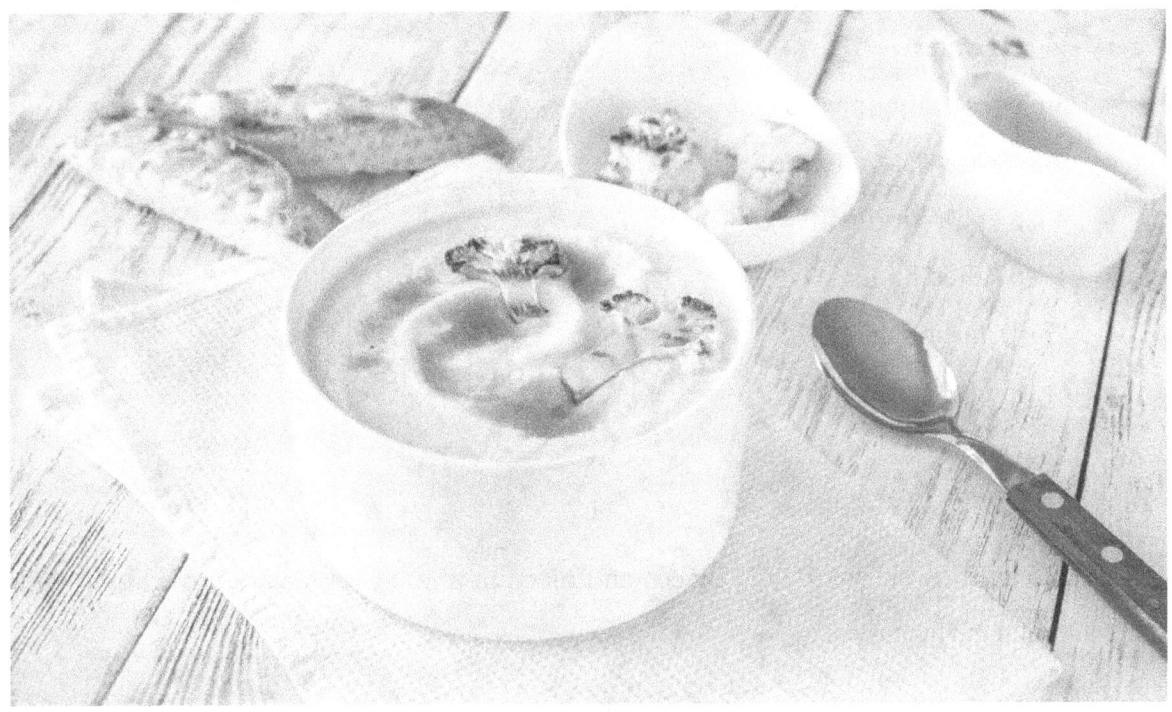

This creamy cauliflower puree is surprisingly tasty and an excellent alternative to mashed potatoes.

Servings: 4

Total Time: 10mins

Ingredients:

- 1 (6-7" diameter) head of cauliflower
- ¼ cup water
- 3 cloves garlic (peeled)
- ⅓ cup low-fat buttermilk
- 4 tsp extra-virgin olive oil (divided)
- 1 tsp salted butter
- ½ tsp garlic salt
- ½ tsp black pepper

Directions:

Break the cauliflower into 2" x2" pieces and place in a microwave-safe bowl along with the water and garlic cloves.

Microwave for 5 minutes, until tender.

Remove the garlic cloves from the bowl, and with a garlic press, crush the cloves and add them to a food processor along with the cooked cauliflower.

Add the buttermilk to the cauliflower, followed by 2 teaspoons of olive oil, salted butter, garlic salt, and black pepper.

In a food blender, process until creamy smooth.

Drizzle the remaining olive oil over the cauliflower puree and enjoy.

Cook's Note: Consult with your surgeon or dietician to make sure this recipe is suitable for your pre or post-bariatric surgery diet plan and or phase.

Green Pea Soup

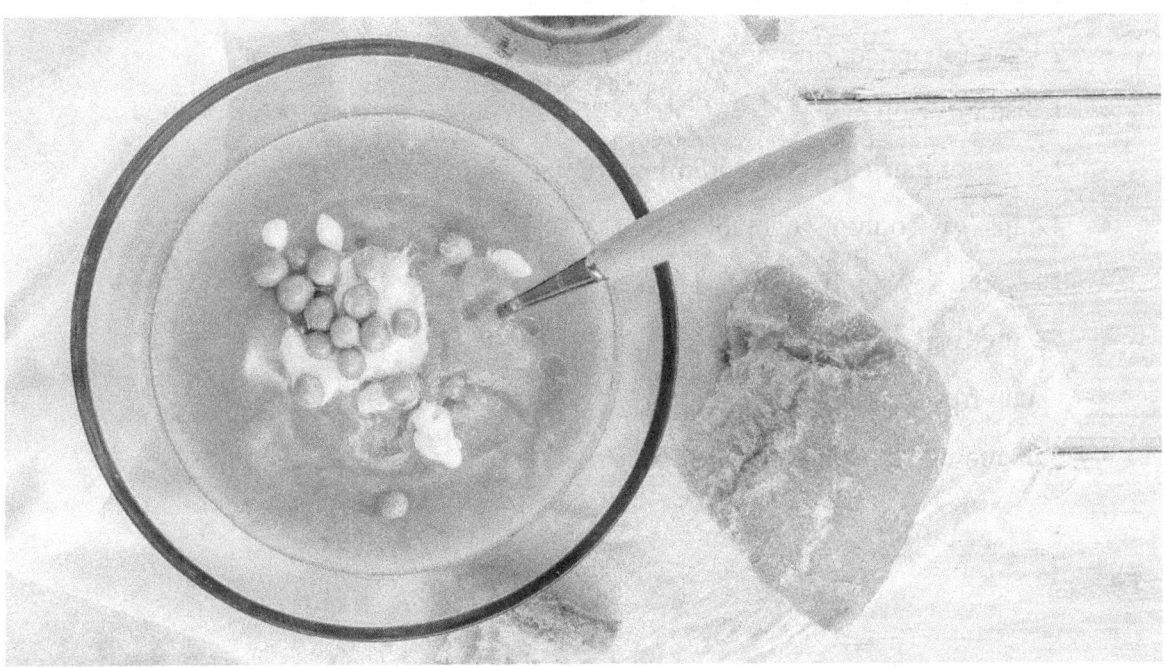

This protein-rich pea soup flavored with fresh mint and parsley is low in calories and gastric bypass or sleeve-friendly for anyone following a puree-only weight loss diet.

Servings: 6

Total Time: 25mins

Ingredients:

- 1 medium onion (peeled and chopped)
- 2 leeks (chopped, rinsed, and drained)
- 1 tbsp olive oil
- 1 clove of garlic (peeled and minced)
- 4 cups low-sodium vegetable stock
- 1 (20-ounce) bag frozen garden peas
- ½ cup fresh mint (chopped)
- ½ cup fresh parsley (chopped)
- Salt and black pepper (to season)

Directions:

In a pan, over moderate heat, sauté the onion and leeks in the olive oil until tender, for 5 minutes.

Stir in the garlic and cook for 60 seconds.

Pour in the vegetable stock and bring to a boil.

Add the frozen peas, and over moderate heat, cook for 3 minutes.

Remove the pan from the heat, and add the mint and parsley, stirring to combine.

Allow the mixture to cool to room temperature for 8-10 minutes.

In a food blender, process the mixture until smooth.

Season the soup with salt and black pepper to taste. You may need to reheat the soup, if necessary.

Cook's Note: Consult with your surgeon or dietician to make sure this recipe is suitable for your pre or post-bariatric surgery diet plan and or phase.

Italian Chicken Puree

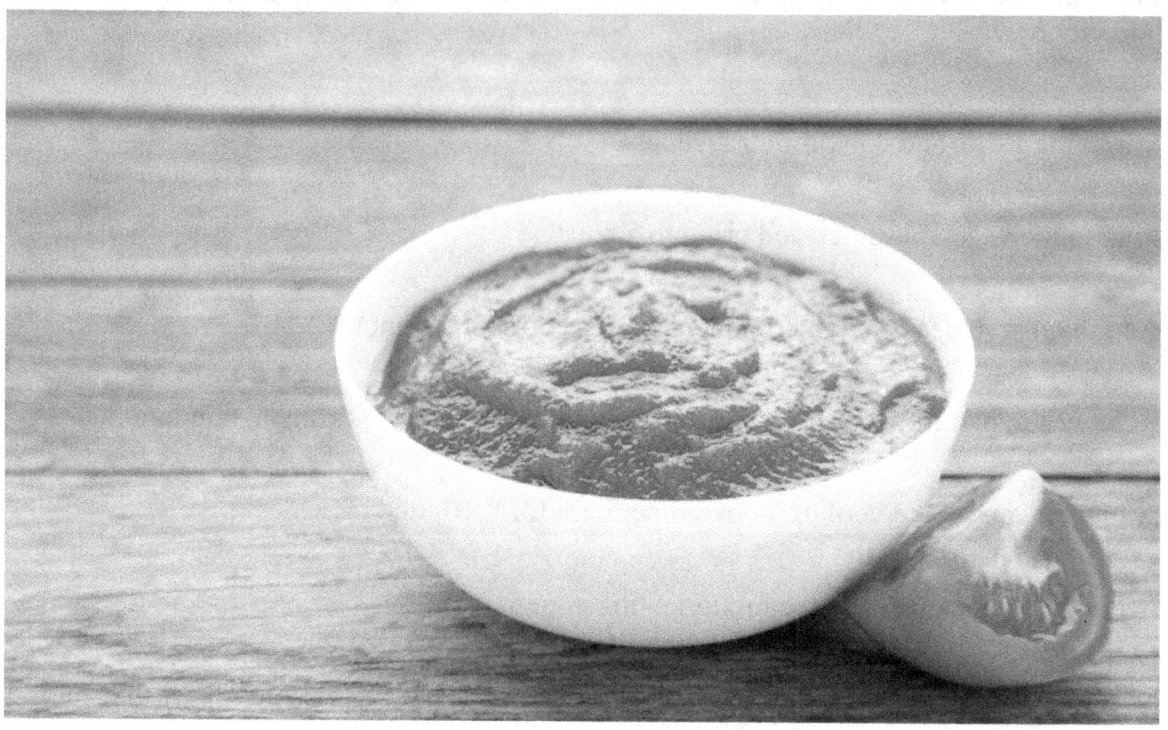

Why compromise on taste when you can enjoy all the flavors of Italian chicken in puree form in a few minutes?

Servings: 1

Total Time: 3mins

Ingredients:

- ¼ cup canned chicken
- 1½ tbsp tomato sauce
- ⅛ tsp salt
- ⅛ tsp black pepper
- 1 tsp Italian seasoning

Directions:

Add the canned chicken, tomato sauce, salt, black pepper, and Italian seasoning to a small food blender until combined and softened.

Transfer to a microwave-safe bowl and microwave for 30 seconds.

Serve and enjoy.

Cook's Note: Consult with your surgeon or dietician to make sure this recipe is suitable for your pre or post-bariatric surgery diet plan and or phase.

Mexican Egg Puree

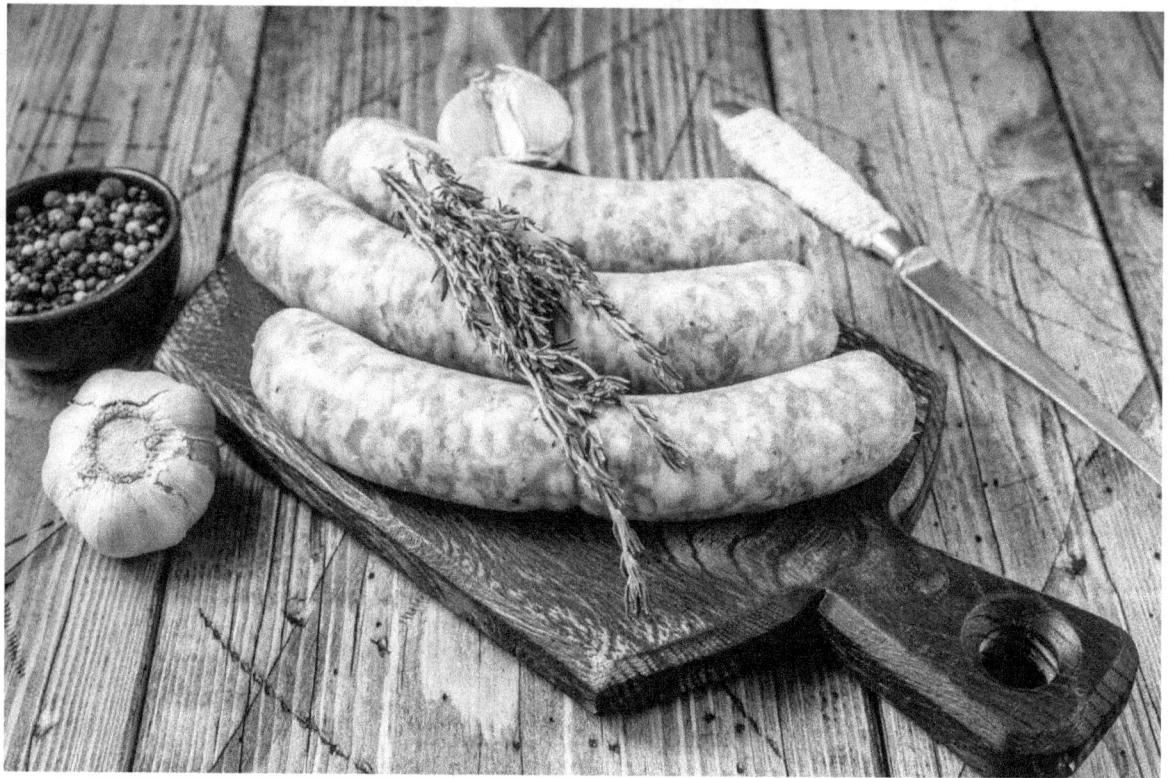

The puréed diet stage post weight loss surgery centers on hydration and protein, and this turkey and egg puree ticks those all-important boxes, texture, and taste.

Servings: 8

Total Time: 15mins

Ingredients:

- 6 eggs
- 1 tbsp full-fat plain Greek yogurt
- 1 tsp cumin
- ½ tsp smoked paprika
- 8 ounces loose turkey sausage
- ¼ cup no-salt-added black beans (drained and rinsed)
- 2 tbsp cilantro (chopped)
- 2 tbsp water

Directions:

In a bowl, whisk the eggs with the yogurt, cumin, and paprika briskly until combined thoroughly. Put the mixture to one side.

In a frying pan, over moderate heat, heat the turkey. Cook the sausage while stirring, using the back of a wooden spoon to break the meat up, for 5-6 minutes or until cooked through.

Turn the heat down to moderate low. Add the egg mixture, moving the ingredients around the pan constantly, and cook for 2-3 minutes.

Stir in the black beans and cook for 60 seconds until warmed through.

Fold in the chopped cilantro and transfer to a food blender along with the water, and pulse until smooth.

Cook's Note: Consult with your surgeon or dietician to make sure this recipe is suitable for your pre or post-bariatric surgery diet plan and or phase.

Pureed Chicken Salad

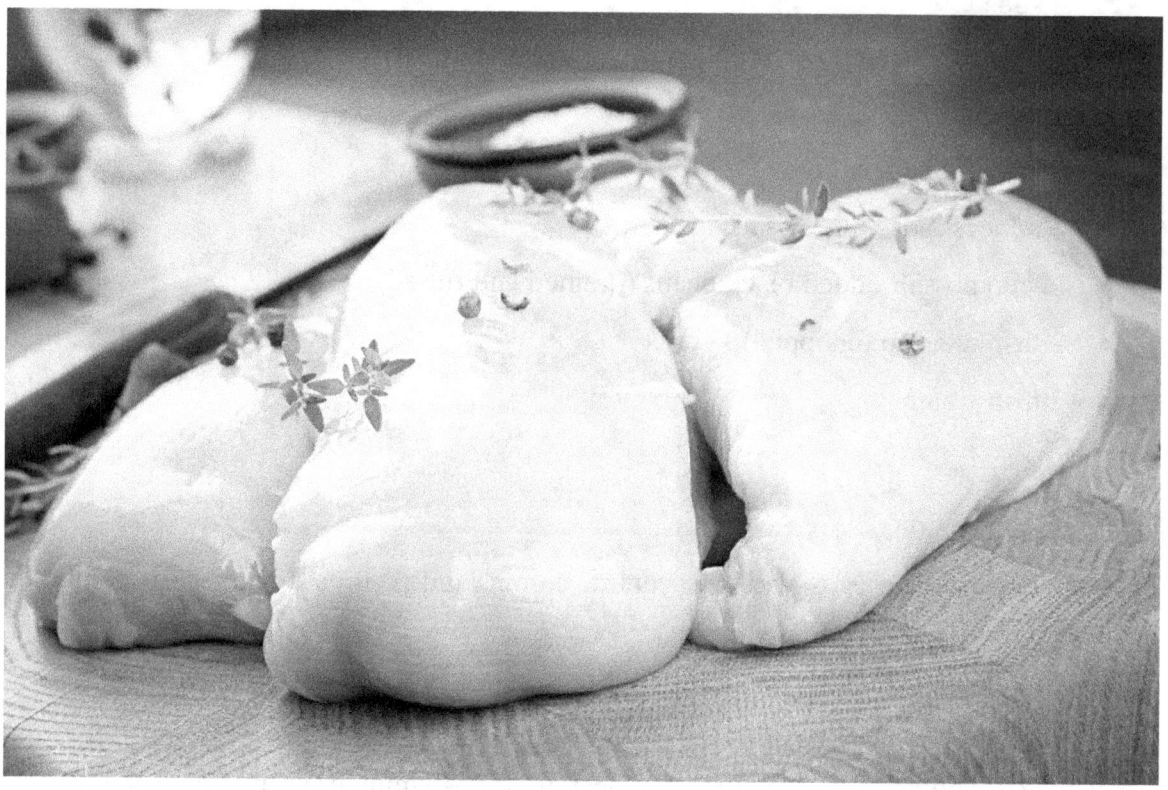

This pureed take on a healthy chicken salad will put you on the road to a speedy recovery and weight loss success.

Servings: 1

Total Time: 4mins

Ingredients:

- 1 skin-free chicken breast (cooked)
- 2 tbsp plain Greek-style yogurt
- 2 tbsp low-fat mayonnaise
- ⅛ tsp celery salt
- ⅛ tsp onion powder
- A dash of black pepper

Directions:

Add the cooked chicken to a food processor, and grind to a fine consistency.

Transfer to a bowl, and stir in the yogurt, mayonnaise, celery salt, and onion powder. Season the mixture with a dash of black pepper, and enjoy.

Cook's Note: Consult with your surgeon or dietician to make sure this recipe is suitable for your pre or post-bariatric surgery diet plan and or phase.

Shepherd-Style Pie

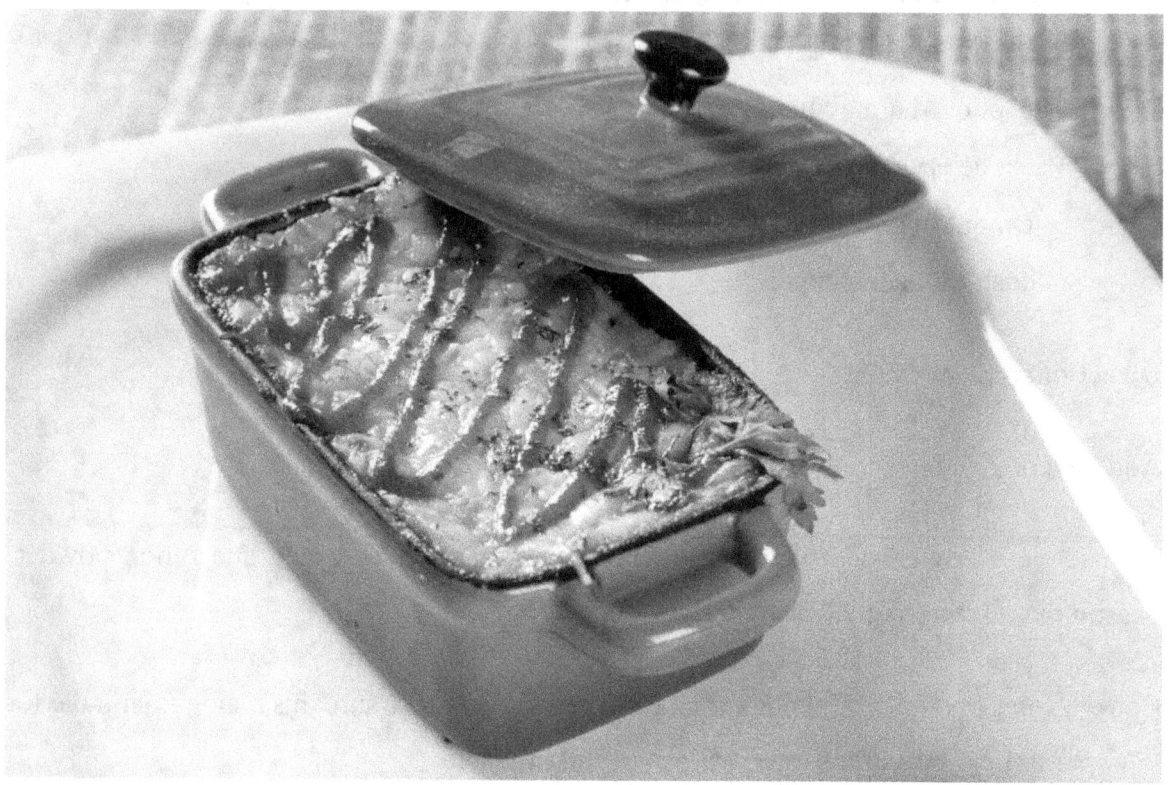

The good thing about this recipe is, the whole family can share and enjoy it too.

Servings: 6

Total Time: 1hour 45mins

Ingredients:

- 1 pound 12 ounces extra-lean ground beef
- 1 large onion (peeled and chopped)
- 2 large carrots
- 1¼ cups passata
- 1 beef stock cube
- 3 tbsp Worcestershire sauce
- Salt and black pepper (to season, optional)
- 1½ pounds rutabagas
- 2 pounds white potatoes

Directions:

Preheat the main oven to 300 degrees F.

On the stovetop, in an ovenproof pan, cook the beef until browned.

Add the onion, carrots and cook until softened, for 5-10 minutes.

Add the passata, crumble in the stock cube, and add the Worcestershire sauce. Season with salt and black pepper and cook for 5 minutes.

Cover with a lid, and cook in the oven for 60 minutes before increasing the oven temperature to 400 degrees F.

In the meantime, in boiling water, cook the rutabaga until softened. Drain and mash the rutabagas to a puree consistency.

At the same time, in a second pan, in boiling water, cook the potatoes until fork-tender. Drain and mash to a puree.

Add the rutabagas to the potatoes and mix to combine.

Transfer the beef mixture to a large casserole dish.

Top the beef with the rutabaga-potato mash.

Bake in the oven for 20-25 minutes, until browned.

Serve and enjoy.

Cook's Note: Consult with your surgeon or dietician to make sure this recipe is suitable for your pre or post-bariatric surgery diet plan and or phase.

Shrimp Puree

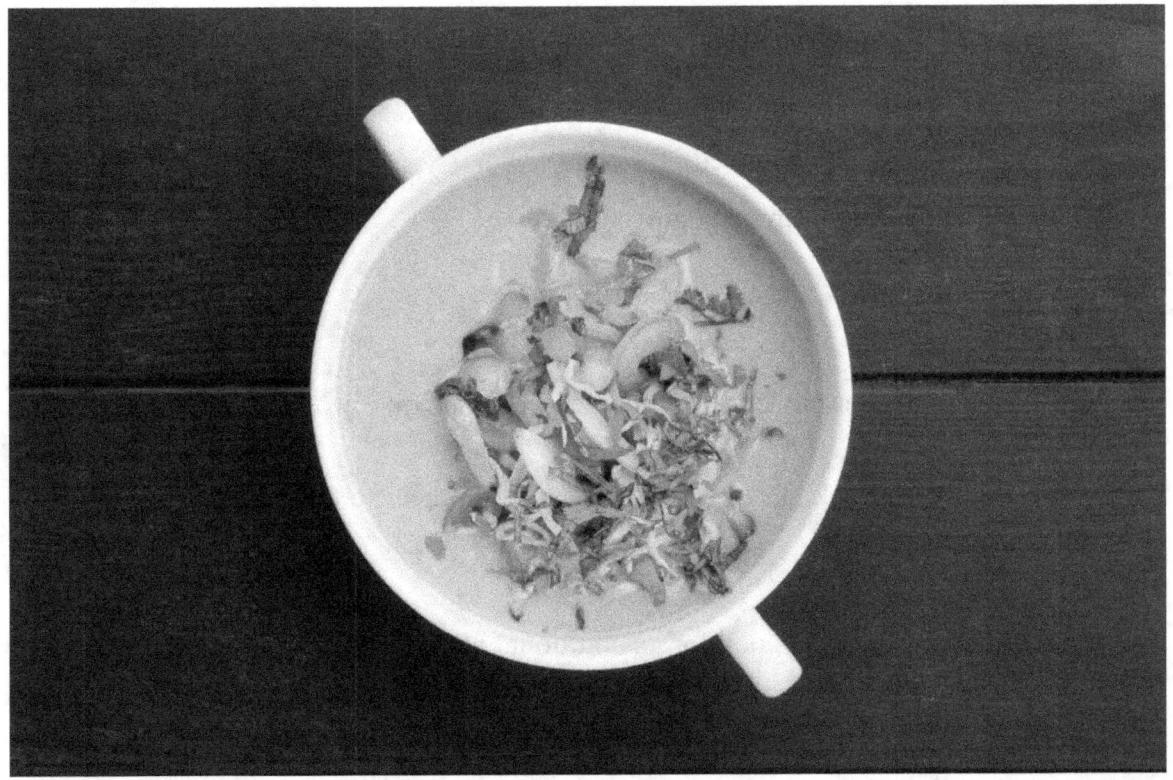

This creamy seafood puree is low on carbs, but it's a real winner when on the protein scale.

Servings: 8-10

Total Time: 10mins

Ingredients:

- 2 tbsp virgin olive oil
- 16 ounces shrimp (peeled and deveined)
- 4 cloves of garlic (peeled and minced)
- ¼ cup fresh parsley (chopped)
- 2 tbsp low-fat, plain Greek yogurt

Directions:

In a large frying pan, over moderate to high heat, heat the oil.

Pat the shrimp dry with a kitchen paper towel and add them to the pan. Cook the shrimp for 2-3 minutes, tossing after 1 minute, until just pink.

To the pan, add the garlic and cook for an additional 60 seconds until fragrant.

Transfer the shrimp to a heatproof bowl, and add the chopped parsley and yogurt, tossing to evenly and well coat.

Transfer the mixture to a food processor and process until silky smooth.

Serve and enjoy.

Cook's Note: Consult with your surgeon or dietician to make sure this recipe is suitable for your pre or post-bariatric surgery diet plan and or phase.

Sweet Potato Casserole

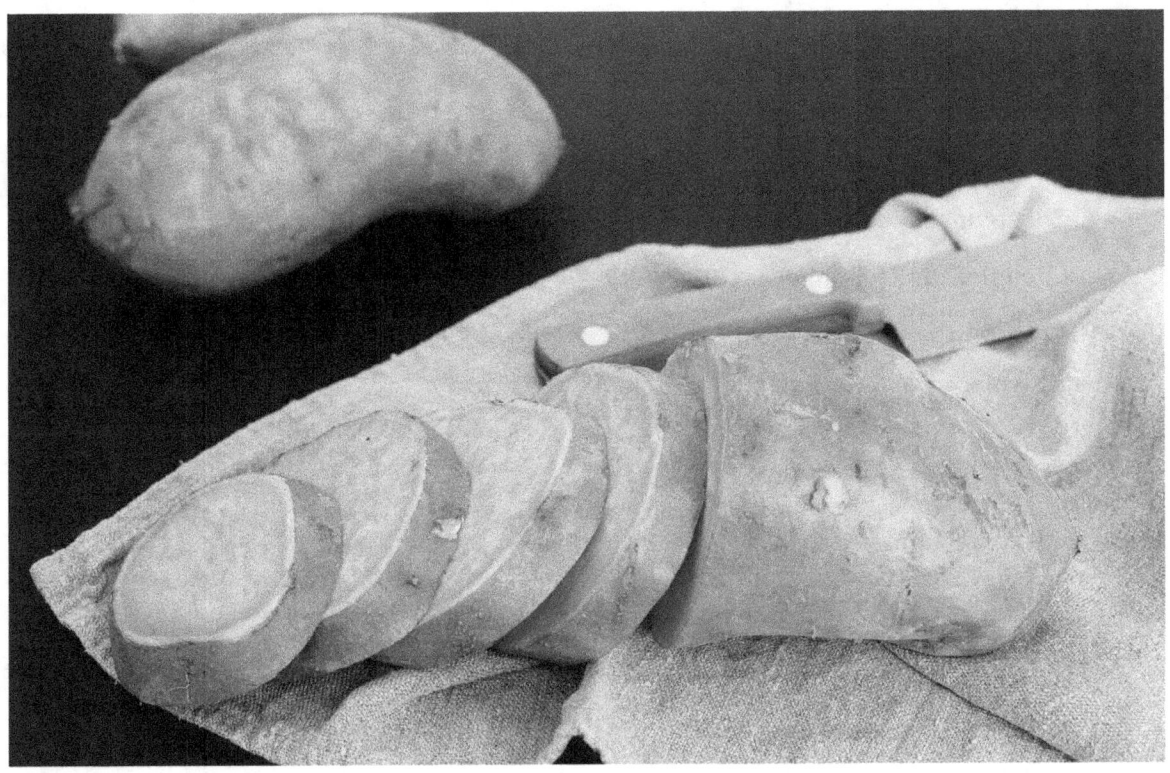

When you are ready to progress from liquids to purees, this sweet potato casserole is ideal. While this veggie isn't a low-carb option, you can add some protein to the recipe and redress the balance.

Servings: 4

Total Time: 30mins

Ingredients:

- 1 large sweet potato (peeled)
- 1 scoop unflavored protein powder
- ¼ tsp pumpkin pie spice
- 1-2 tbsp sugar and calorie-free sweetener
- 2 tbsp unsalted butter
- ½ cup pecans (chopped)
- ⅛ tsp salt

Directions:

Preheat the main oven to 350 degrees F.

Bring a pot of water to a boil.

Add the sweet potato to the pot and boil for 8-10 minutes, until fork-tender.

In a bowl, mash the cooked potato well before adding the protein powder, calorie-free sweetener, pumpkin pie spice, and mash once more. You can also do this using an immersion blender.

Spoon the mash into ramekins.

In a small pan, melt the butter. Stir in the pecans and season with salt, tossing to ensure the nuts are evenly and well coated.

Top the ramekins with the pecan mixture and bake in the preheated oven for 12-15 minutes, until toasted.

Cook's Note: Consult with your surgeon or dietician to make sure this recipe is suitable for your pre or post-bariatric surgery diet plan and or phase.

Tuna Mornay

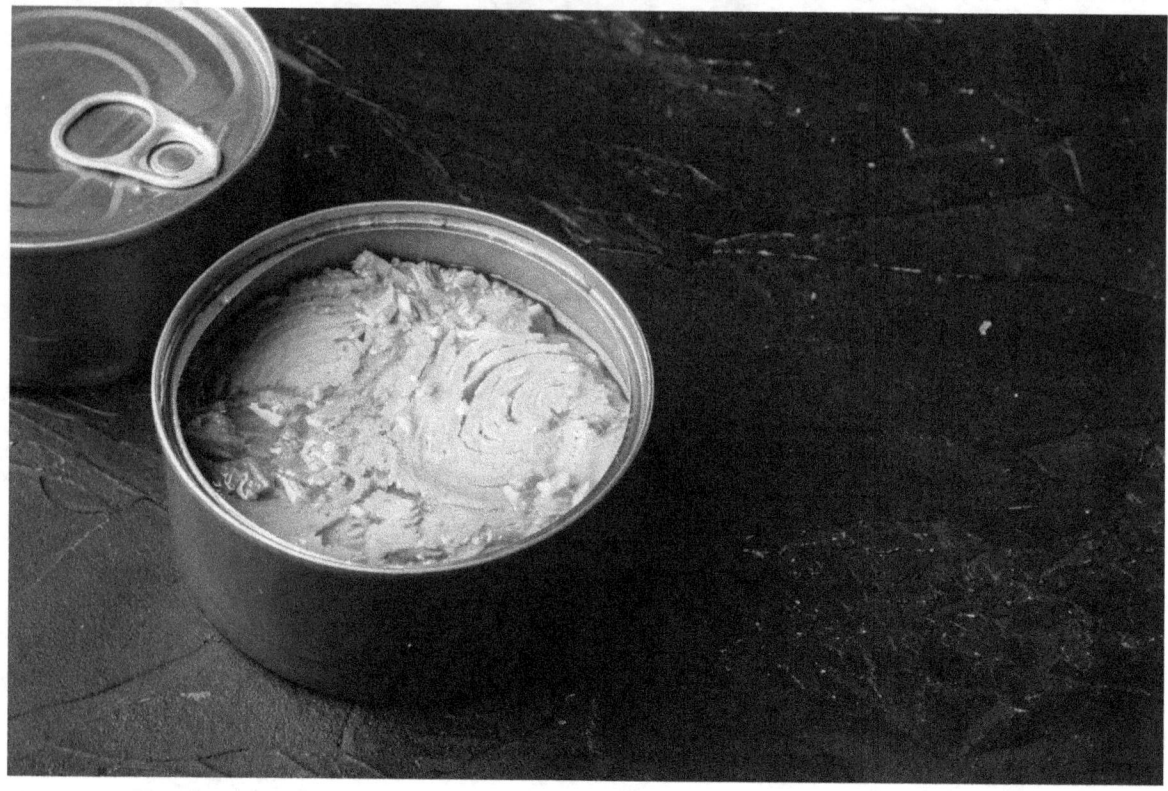

Canned tuna is rich in protein, vitamins, and minerals. It also contains omega-3, and this recipe is perfect for both the puree and soft food steps to recovery.

Servings: 4

Total Time: 18mins

Ingredients:

- Nonstick zero-calorie cooking spray oil
- 1 brown onion (peeled and chopped)
- 1 large celery stalk (trimmed and finely chopped)
- ¼ cup plain flour
- 2 cups low fat milk
- 14 ounces canned tuna in spring water (drained and flaked)
- ⅔ cup reduced-fat cheese (grated)
- Fresh parsley (chopped)

Directions:

Using nonstick cooking spray, spritz a pan and cook the onion and celery.

Add the flour, and stir for 60 seconds. Take the pan off the heat and gradually add the milk while stirring continually.

Return the pan to the heat, and stir until the sauce thickens.

Take the pan off the heat, and stir in the canned tuna and grated cheese.

Remove from the heat, and in a food blender, puree the mixture.

Garnish with parsley and serve.

Cook's Note: Consult with your surgeon or dietician to make sure this recipe is suitable for your pre or post-bariatric surgery diet plan and or phase.

Phase 3: Soft Foods

Avocado Egg Salad

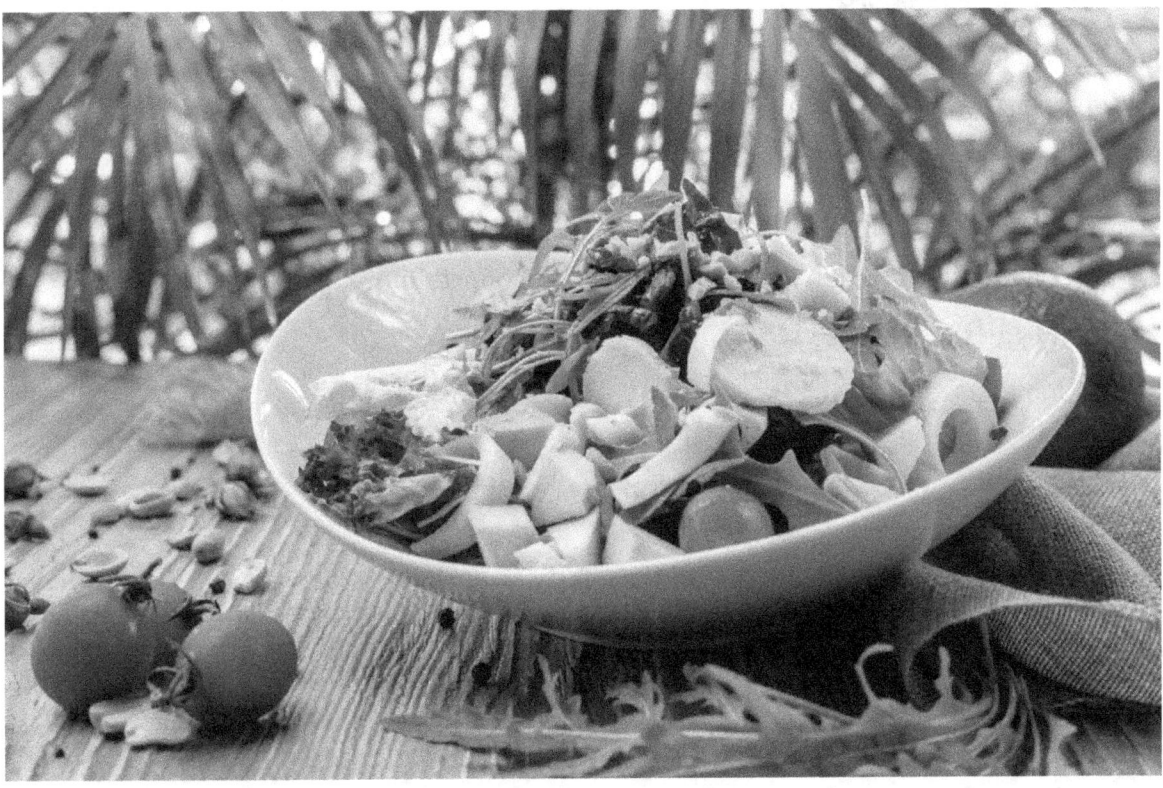

Eggs are an excellent protein source, and this recipe is the perfect texture for the soft phase following bariatric surgery.

Servings: 4

Total Time: 8mins

Ingredients:

- 4 hard-boiled eggs
- 1 tbsp dill pickle relish
- 3 tbsp reduced-fat mayonnaise
- 1 tsp onion powder
- Salt and black pepper (to season)
- 1 large ripe avocado (peeled, pitted, and chopped into bite-size pieces)
- Veggies (cooked, to serve)
- Paprika (to garnish)

Directions:

Peel and slice the hard-boiled eggs, and carefully remove the yolks.

In a bowl, combine the yolks with the dill pickle relish, mayonnaise, and onion powder. Season the mixture with salt and black pepper.

Thoroughly chop the egg white and add the chopped avocado.

Spoon the mayo mixture over the top, and mix gently to combine.

Serve the egg salad on its own or with soft veggies.

Garnish with paprika and enjoy.

Cook's Note: Consult with your surgeon or dietician to make sure this recipe is suitable for your pre or post-bariatric surgery diet plan and or phase.

Baked Fish with Almond Chutney

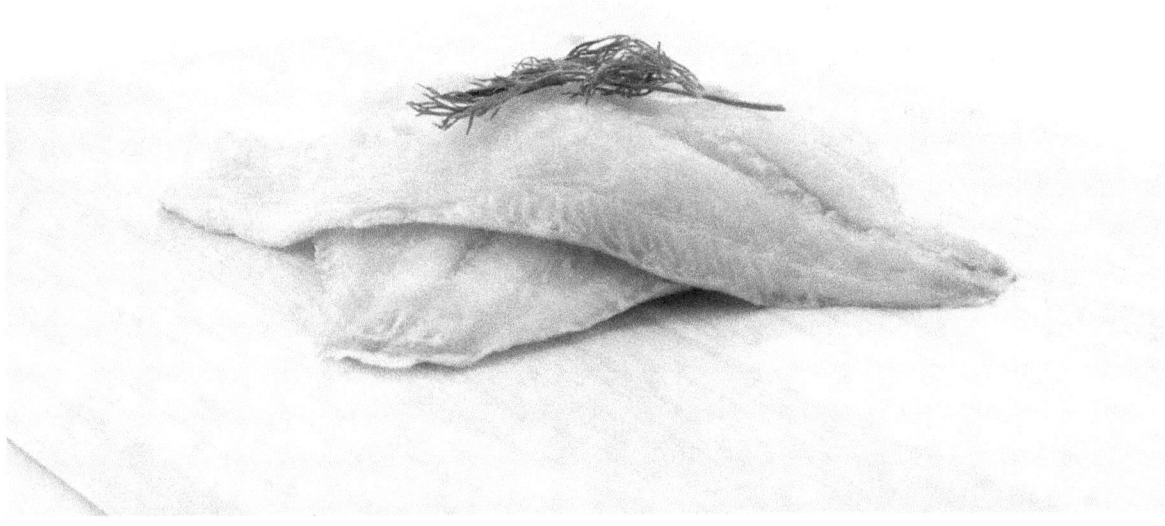

Just because you have had bariatric surgery doesn't mean that you can't enjoy flavorful food, and this fish dish topped with homemade almond chutney will have everyone asking for more.

Servings: 8

Total Time: 30mins

Ingredients:

- 1 tbsp olive oil
- 2 tsp freshly squeezed lemon juice
- 16 ounces white fish fillets (of choice)
- ½ cup almonds (sliced)
- ½ cup no-salt-added diced tomatoes
- 1 tsp coriander

Directions:

Preheat the main oven to 375 degrees F.

In a large baking dish, whisk the oil with the fresh lemon juice.

Using a kitchen paper towel, pat the fish dry.

In a single layer, lay the fish in the baking dish and turn over to coat in the oil and juice.

Transfer to the oven for 15-20 minutes until the fish is cooked through. The actual cooking time will depend on the thickness of the fish.

In a food processor, combine the almonds with tomatoes and coriander. Pulse the mixture to chop and incorporate. The mixture is ready when it's chunky.

Take the fish out of the oven.

Pour the chutney over the surface of the fish, and return it to the oven until warm, for 2-3 minutes.

Cook's Note: Consult with your surgeon or dietician to make sure this recipe is suitable for your pre or post-bariatric surgery diet plan and or phase.

Cottage Cheese Bake

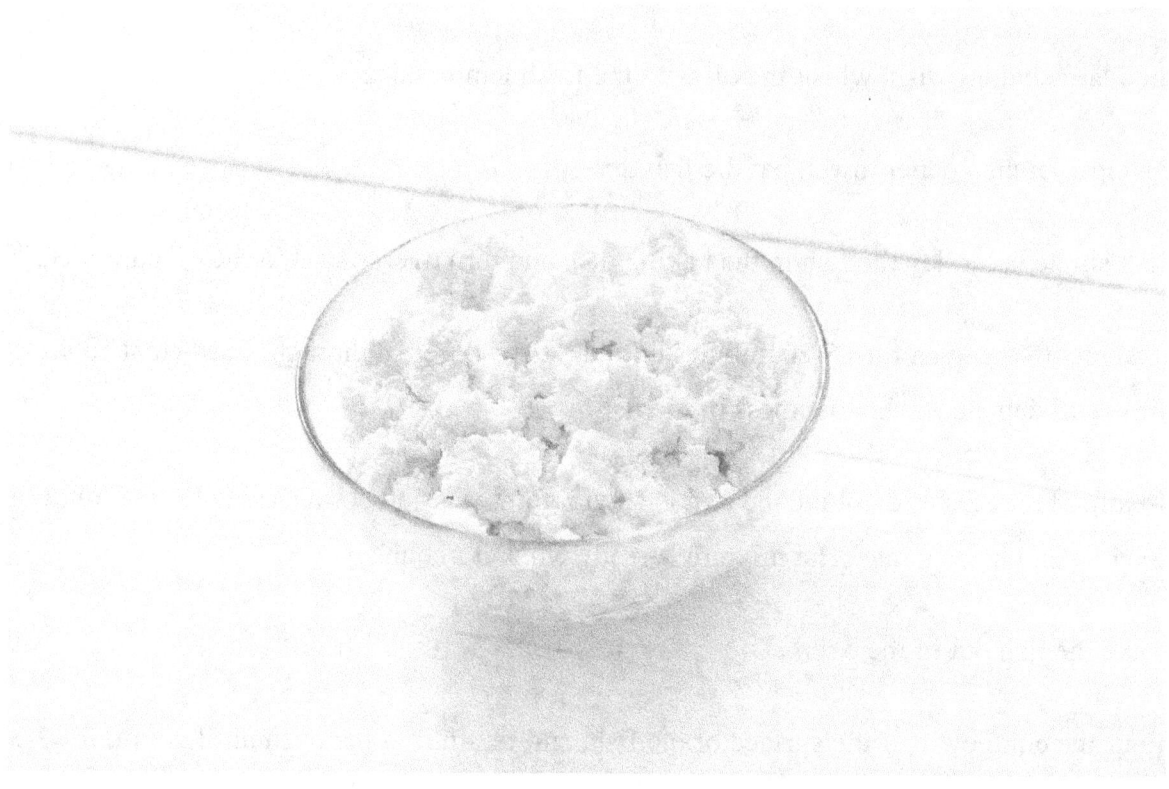

Cottage cheese is a great choice for anyone in the soft food phase of their diet plan following gastric bypass or sleeve surgery. A half-cup serving of 4 percent cottage cheese provides 12-14 grams of protein.

Servings: 8

Total Time: 30mins

Ingredients:

- 2 cups reduced-fat plain cottage cheese
- 2 eggs
- 10 ounces frozen spinach (thawed and well-drained)
- ½ cup Parmesan cheese (grated)
- Sea salt and freshly ground black pepper

Directions:

Preheat the main oven to 350 degrees F.

In a bowl, combine the cottage cheese with the eggs, spinach, and Parmesan cheese.

Spoon the mixture into an 8" square pan and bake in the oven until the cheese bubbles, for 25-30 minutes.

Remove from the oven and allow to rest for 5 minutes.

Season the bake with sea salt and freshly ground black pepper and enjoy.

Cook's Note: Consult with your surgeon or dietician to make sure this recipe is suitable for your pre or post-bariatric surgery diet plan and or phase.

Greek-Style Turkey Burgers with Homemade Tzatziki Sauce

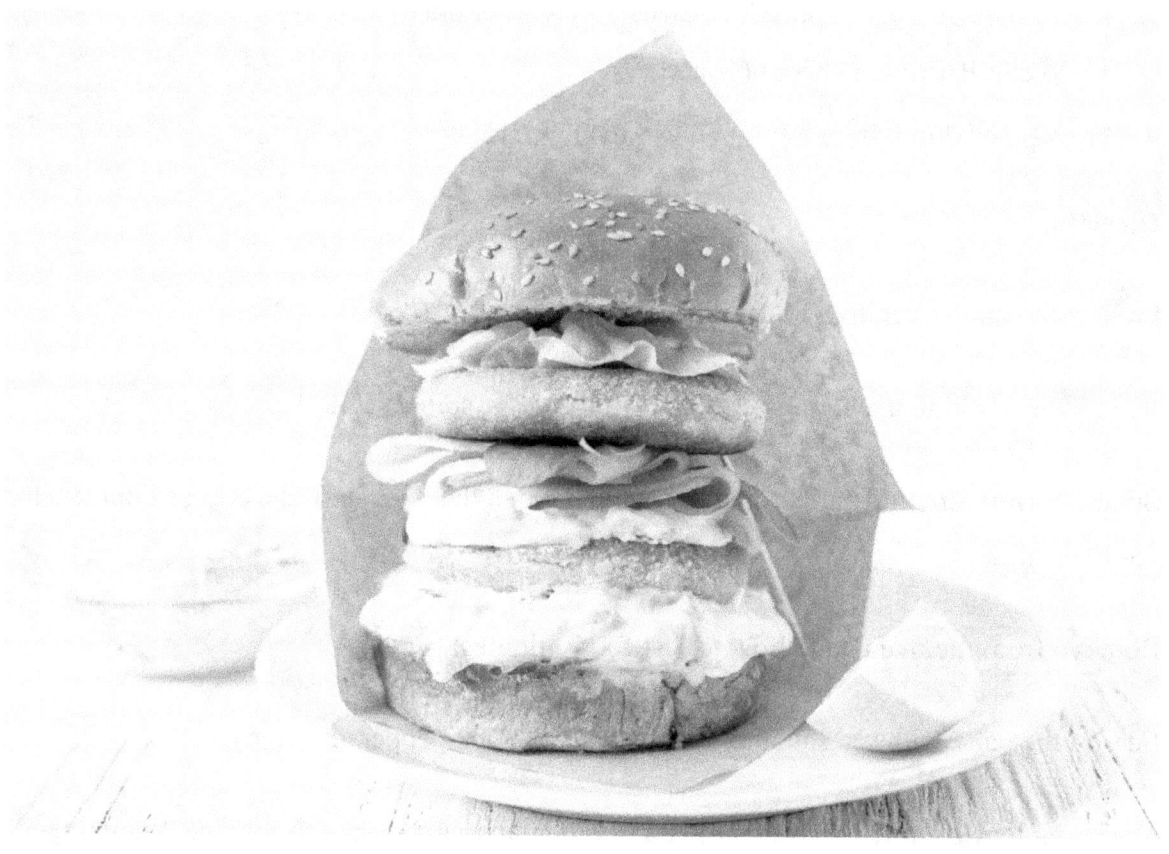

These Greek-style turkey burgers are proof positive that soft food never tasted so good!

Servings: 4

Total Time: 30mins

Ingredients:

- ¼ cup red onion (peeled and sliced)
- ¼ cup mushrooms (sliced)
- ¼ cup red bell peppers (sliced)
- ¼ tsp salt
- ¼ cup fresh basil leaves
- 2 cloves garlic (peeled)
- ¼ tsp black pepper
- 1 pound extra-lean ground turkey
- Nonstick cooking spray
- 4 slices fresh pineapple

Tzatziki:

- ½ cup cucumber (peeled, seeded, and finely sliced)
- 1 cup plain Greek yogurt
- 1 tbsp freshly squeezed lemon juice
- ¼ tsp salt
- 1 clove of garlic (peeled and left whole)

Directions:

Preheat your grill.

In a food processor, combine the slices of red onion, sliced mushrooms, red bell pepper slices, basil leaves, garlic, salt, and black pepper. Cover with a lid, and pulse until chopped finely.

Add the onion mixture to the ground turkey in a bowl.

Using clean hands, mix until combined and form the mixture into 4 even-sized, moist patties.

Spritz aluminum foil with nonstick cooking spray.

Arrange the patties on the foil, and transfer to the preheated grill, cooking for 5-6 minutes on each side, until the juices run clear and the meat is no longer pink.

Place the slices of fresh pineapple on the grill and cook for approximately 4-5 minutes on each side.

For the tzatziki: In a food processor, combine the cucumber with the Greek yogurt, lemon juice, salt, and garlic clove. Cover and process until combined. Transfer the tzatziki to the fridge until needed.

To serve: Top the turkey patties with the pineapple and a dollop of tzatziki.

Cook's Note: Consult with your surgeon or dietician to make sure this recipe is suitable for your pre or post-bariatric surgery diet plan and or phase.

Instant Pot Turkey Chili

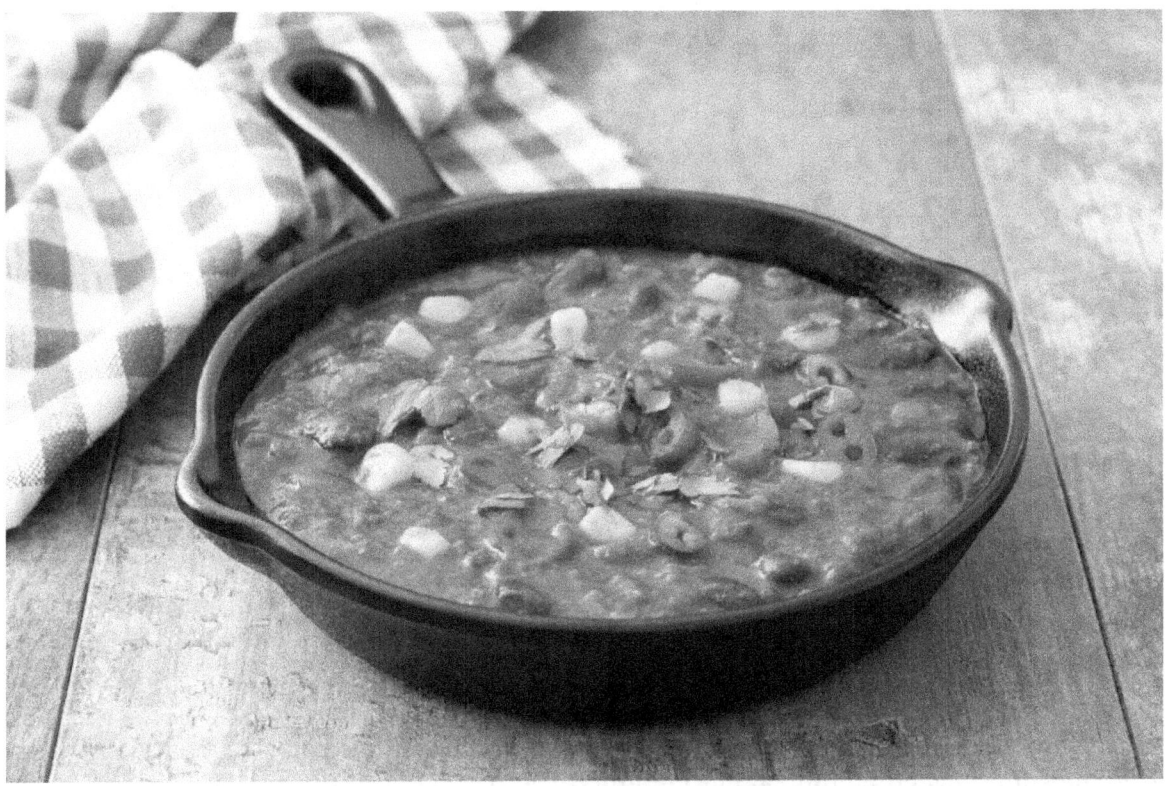

Most of us like a good chili now and again, and just because you have undergone bariatric surgery doesn't mean you can't still enjoy this favorite family meal.

Servings: 6

Total Time: 25mins

Ingredients:

- 2 tbsp olive oil
- 1 onion (peeled and chopped)
- 1½ tbsp chili powder
- 1½ tsp cumin
- 16 ounces lean ground turkey
- 2 (14-ounce) cans crushed tomatoes
- 1 cup low-sodium chicken broth
- 1 (14-ounce) can red kidney beans (rinsed and drained)
- Salt and black pepper

Directions:

Using an Instant Pot, and on the sauté function, heat the olive oil, add the onion, and cook until softened.

Add the chili powder, cumin, and ground turkey and sauté until the meat is browned.

Stir in the canned tomatoes and add the chicken broth, close the pot's lid, and on high cook for 10 minutes.

When cooked, release the valve, stir in the red kidney beans. Season the chili with salt and black pepper and either serve as is or puree.

Cook's Note: Consult with your surgeon or dietician to make sure this recipe is suitable for your pre or post-bariatric surgery diet plan and or phase.

Quinoa Muffins

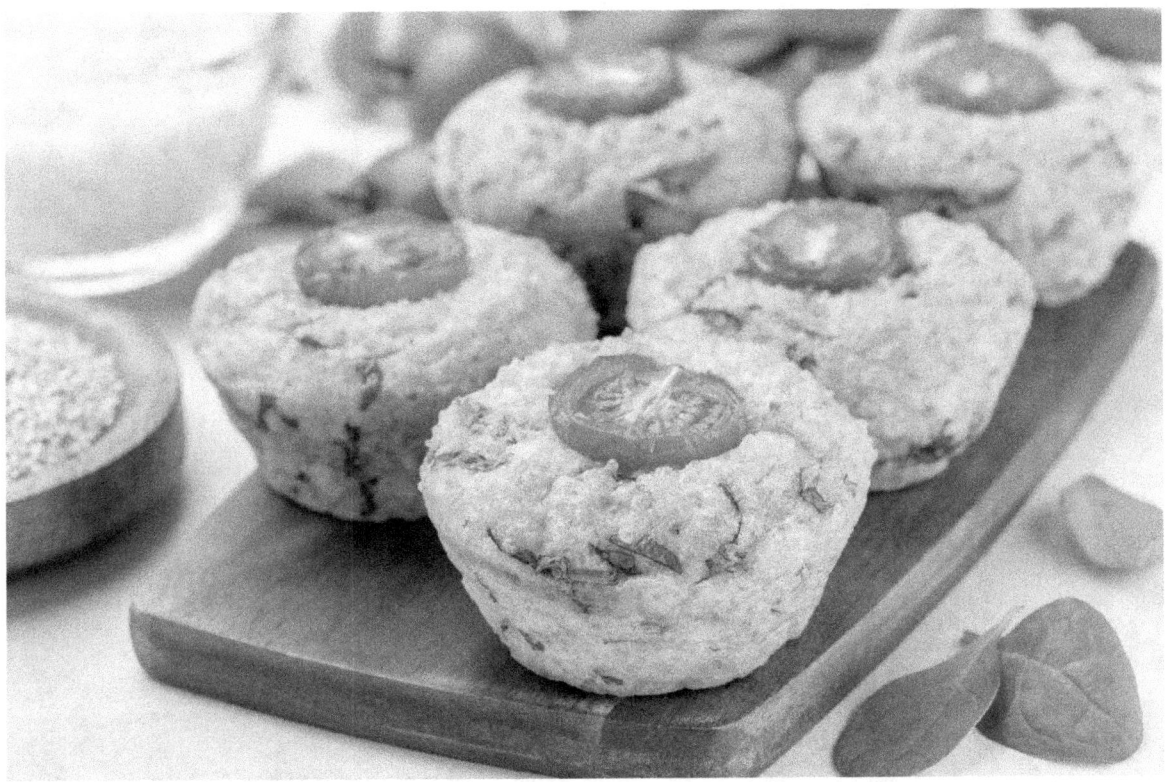

It's time to give whole grains a chance to shine! And what better way is there than baking up a batch of these savory quinoa muffins?

Servings: 24

Total Time: 40mins

Ingredients:

- Nonstick baking spray
- 2 large eggs
- ¼ cup canola oil
- 1½ tsp baking powder
- ¼ cup skim milk
- 2 cups flour
- 1 tsp salt
- ½ tsp finely ground black pepper
- 4 cups cooked quinoa (cooled)
- ½ cup frozen peas (thawed)
- 1 cup fresh spinach (chopped)
- 1 zucchini (grated)
- 1 tsp fresh dill (chopped)
- ½ cup reduced-fat feta (crumbled)

Directions:

Preheat the main oven to 350 degrees F.

Spritz 2 (12-cup) muffin pans with nonstick baking spray.

In a bowl, whisk the eggs with the canola oil and skim milk.

In a second, smaller bowl, whisk the flour, salt, baking powder, and black pepper.

Stir in the cooked and cooled quinoa.

Pour the mixture into the wet ingredients, stirring until incorporated but taking care not to over-mix.

Next, add peas, spinach, zucchini, dill, and feta. Stir the mixture until just incorporated.

Spoon the mixture into the muffin pans and bake in the preheated oven for 25-30 minutes, until springy to the touch.

Cook's Note: Consult with your surgeon or dietician to make sure this recipe is suitable for your pre or post-bariatric surgery diet plan and or phase.

Tilapia Stuffed Mushrooms

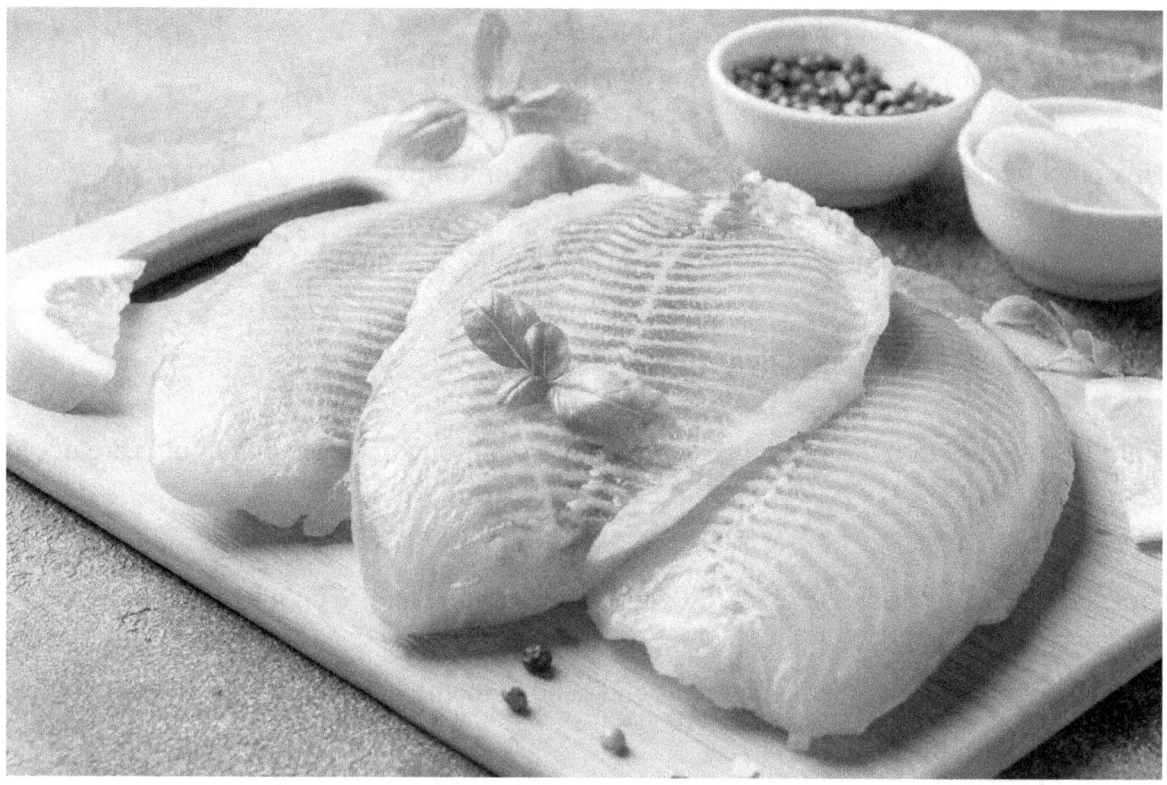

It's always a good idea to create recipes that the whole family can share. Just because they are soft food doesn't mean that everyone can't enjoy these fish-stuffed mushrooms!

Servings: 4

Total Time: 55mins

Ingredients:

- Nonstick cooking spray
- 2 (16-ounce) packages Portobello mushrooms (wiped clean and stemmed)
- 1 tbsp olive oil
- ⅛ cup low-fat butter substitute
- 1 large sweet onion (peeled and diced)
- 1 medium green bell pepper (diced)
- 1 medium red bell pepper (diced)
- 1 medium zucchini (diced)
- 1 tbsp onion powder
- 1 tbsp garlic powder
- ½ tsp Old Bay seasoning
- 1 tbsp freshly squeezed lemon juice
- 1 large egg
- 2 scoops unflavored protein powder
- 4 fillets of tilapia (pre-cooked)
- 2 cups Swiss cheese (shredded and divided)
- Salt and black pepper

Directions:

Preheat the main oven to 400 degrees F.

Spray a baking sheet with nonstick cooking spray.

Arrange the mushroom caps on the baking sheet, gill side facing upwards.

Over high heat, in a nonstick frying pan, heat the olive oil and butter substitute until the butter melts.

Add the onions, green and red bell peppers, zucchini, onion powder, garlic powder, and Old Bay seasoning. Over moderate heat, sauté for approximately 5 minutes, until the veggies are fork-tender and the onions translucent. At the very end of cooking, stir in the fresh lemon juice.

Remove the pan from the heat and allow the veggies to cool for a minimum of 8-10 minutes.

In a bowl, beat the egg. Whisk in the unflavored protein powder.

Break the fillets of cooked fish into small size pieces. Add the fish to the egg.

Stir in the veggie mixture followed by 1 cup of Swiss cheese to combine.

Spoon the mixture into each mushroom cup until filled.

Season with salt and black pepper.

Bake the mushrooms in the preheated oven for 15-20 minutes until cooked.

Remove the pan from the oven and top each mushroom with a scattering of the remaining Swiss cheese.

Return the pan to the oven for an additional 5 minutes until the cheese melts, and enjoy warm.

Cook's Note: Consult with your surgeon or dietician to make sure this recipe is suitable for your pre or post-bariatric surgery diet plan and or phase.

Tofu Scramble

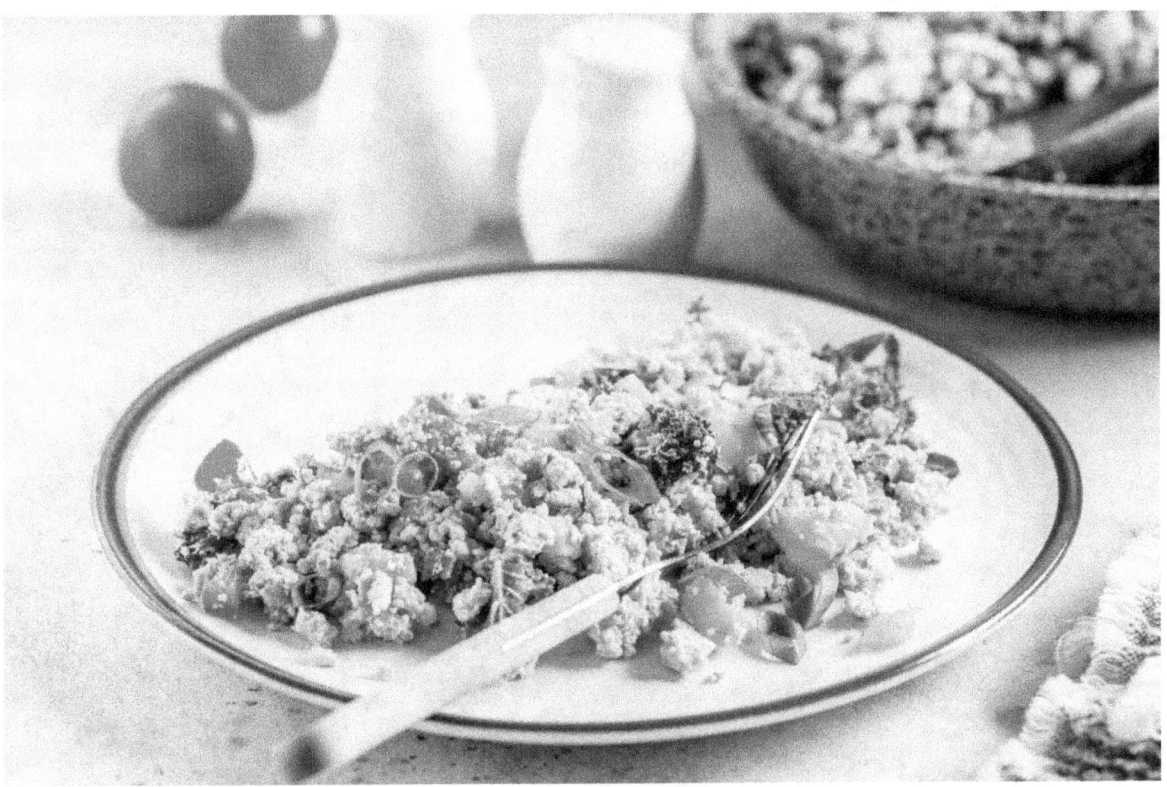

Tofu scramble is a great alternative to eggs for breakfast. Just half a cup of tofu will give you around 12 grams of protein which is very important when it comes to weight loss.

Servings: 4

Total Time: 20mins

Ingredients:

- 1 tbsp olive oil
- ¼ cup onion (peeled and diced)
- 1 whole red bell pepper (diced)
- 3 cloves garlic (peeled and minced)
- 4 slice ripe avocado (to serve)
- 1 cup kale
- 1 (16-ounce) block firm tofu
- 1 tbsp low-sodium soy sauce

Directions:

Over moderate heat in a pan, heat the oil. Add the onions and red bell peppers and sauté until softened.

Next, add the garlic and sauté for an additional 60 seconds.

Stir in the kale, cover with a lid, and allow to steam until wilted.

Add the tofu to a bowl, followed by the soy sauce. Using a fork, mash until scrambled, and no chunks remain.

Remove the lid from the pan, turn the heat up to high and add the scrambled tofu mixture. Stir well and allow to sit for 3-4 minutes. Flip the tofu scrambled over and allow to rest for an additional 3-4 minutes until browned.

Serve each portion of a scramble with a slice of ripe avocado and enjoy.

Cook's Note: Consult with your surgeon or dietician to make sure this recipe is suitable for your pre or post-bariatric surgery diet plan and or phase.

Tuna Zoodle Casserole

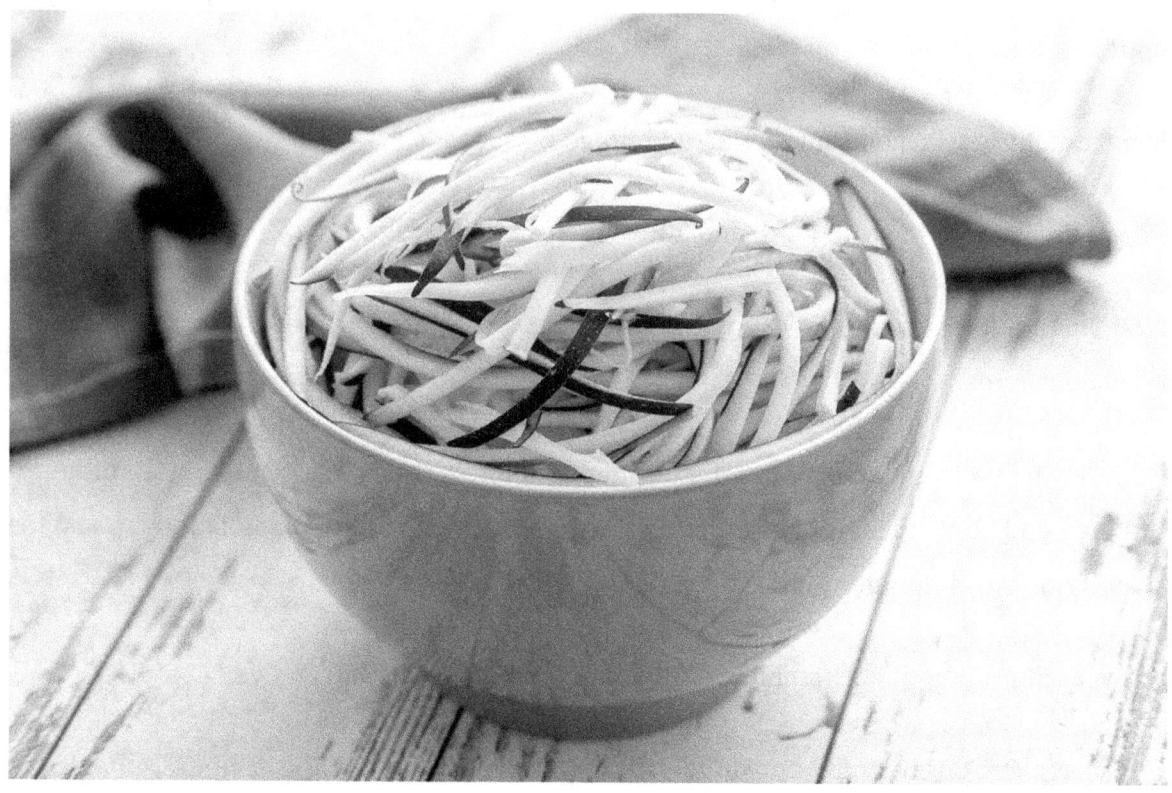

Spiralized zucchini is a healthy alternative to carb-laden pasta, and what's more, you won't even notice the difference.

Servings: 2-3

Total Time: 35mins

Ingredients:

- Nonstick cooking spray
- ½ small onion (peeled and diced)
- 4 ounces canned pea and carrot mix (drained)
- 4 ounces tuna in spring water (drained)
- 6 ounces reduced-fat cream of mushroom soup (undiluted)
- 1 medium-size zucchini (spiralized)
- ½ tbsp butter
- ⅓ cup whole wheat breadcrumbs optional
- 2 tbsp Parmesan cheese (grated)

Directions:

Preheat the main oven to 350 degrees F.

Spritz a skillet with nonstick cooking spray and set on the stovetop over moderate heat. Add the onion to the pan and sauté until tender, for 2-3 minutes.

Add the canned peas and carrots, drained tuna, and mushroom soup to the pan. Heat for another 2-3 minutes, stirring until combined.

Add the spiralized zucchini noodles and stir to combine. Transfer the mixture to a small baking dish.

In a microwave-safe bowl, in the microwave, melt the butter. Add the breadcrumbs to the melted butter stir to incorporate.

Spoon the breadcrumb mixture over the top, followed by the Parmesan cheese, and bake in the preheated oven for 25-30 minutes or until the topping is crisp.

Serve and enjoy.

Cook's Note: Consult with your surgeon or dietician to make sure this recipe is suitable for your pre or post-bariatric surgery diet plan and or phase.

Turkey Bacon, Egg and Cheese Muffins

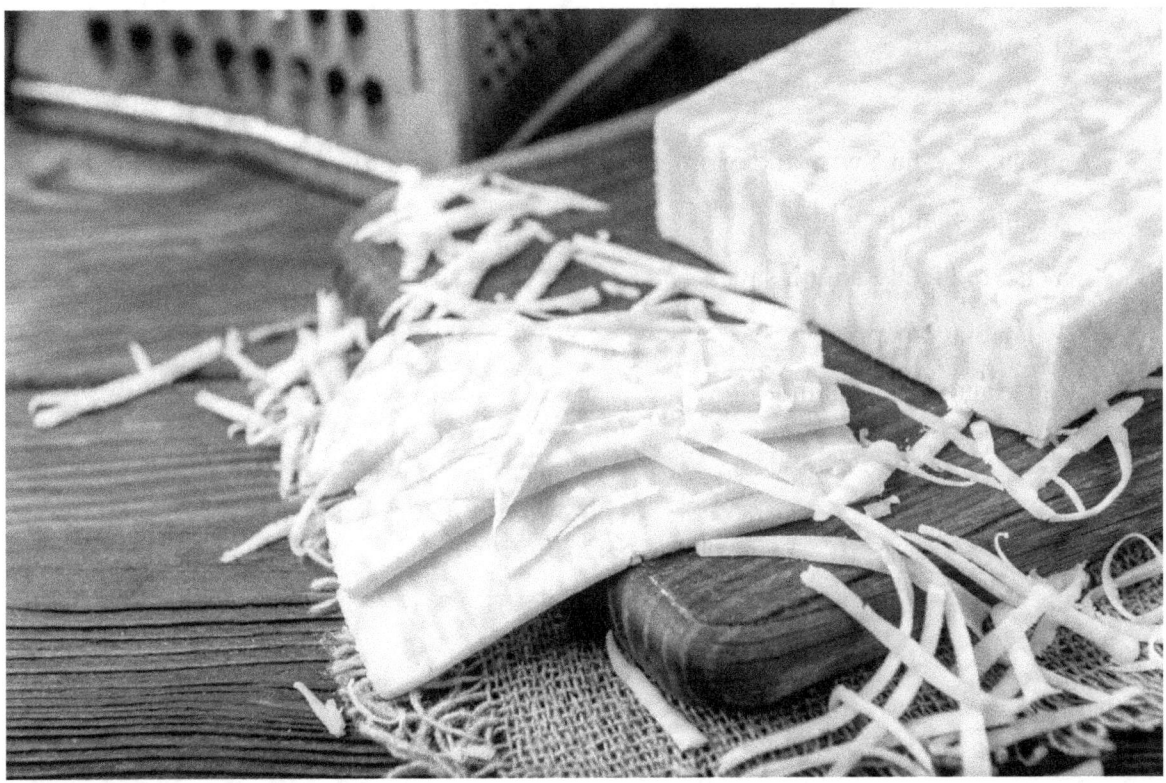

These light and fluffy muffins are low-calorie, low in fat, but high in protein. They are ideal for breakfast, brunch or to pop in your lunchbox.

Servings: 12

Total Time: 30mins

Ingredients:

- Nonstick baking spray
- 12 slices turkey bacon (cooked and sliced into thirds)
- 6 large eggs
- ¾ cup low-fat Swiss and Monterey Jack cheese blend (shredded and divided)
- ½ cup 1% milk
- ¼ tsp reduced-sodium salt
- ¼ tsp black pepper
- ¼ tsp Italian seasoning

Directions:

Preheat the main oven to 350 degrees F. Spritz a 12-cup muffin pan with nonstick cooking spray.

Place 3 strips of cooked turkey bacon to the bottom of each muffin cup. Set the muffin pan aside.

In a mixing bowl, combine the eggs with ½ cup of the cheese blend, milk, salt, black pepper, and Italian seasoning. Mix thoroughly to incorporate.

Pour the mixture into the muffin cups.

Scatter the remaining cheese blend over the 12 muffin cups and bake in the oven for 20-25 minutes until the eggs are entirely set.

Remove from the oven, and enjoy.

Cook's Note: Consult with your surgeon or dietician to make sure this recipe is suitable for your pre or post-bariatric surgery diet plan and or phase.

Phase 4: Stabilizing Foods

Baked Marinara Chicken

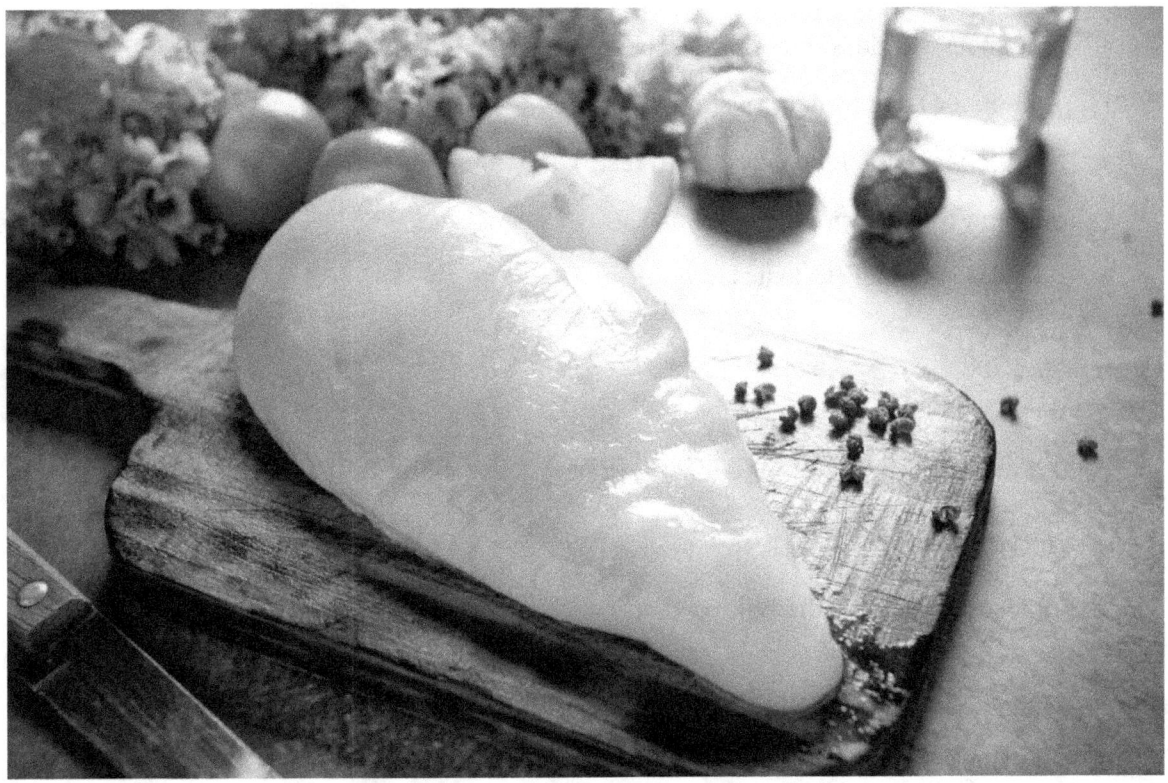

You have successfully reached the stabilizing stage so reward yourself with this Italian-style chicken and a serving of your favorite steamed veggies.

Servings: 4

Total Time: 1hour15mins

Ingredients:

- Nonstick cooking spray
- 16 ounces skinless, boneless chicken breast
- 1 (6-ounce) can tomato paste
- Splash of apple cider vinegar (to taste)
- Salt and black pepper (to season)
- Italian seasoning (to taste)

Directions:

Preheat the main oven to 350 degrees F. Spritz a 9x13" baking dish with nonstick cooking spray.

Lay the chicken breasts in the baking dish.

Add the tomato paste to a small bowl. Fill the empty can of tomato paste with water, add to the bowl, and stir to combine.

Season to taste with a splash of apple cider vinegar, salt, black pepper, and Italian seasoning.

Spoon an equal amount of the mixture over the chicken evenly to cover.

Bake in the preheated oven until the meat registers an internal temperature of 165 degrees F. This step will take approximately 60 minutes.

Remove from the oven before serving with fresh veggies of choice.

Cook's Note: Consult with your surgeon or dietician to make sure this recipe is suitable for your pre or post-bariatric surgery diet plan and or phase.

Beef Stew with Apricots and Saffron

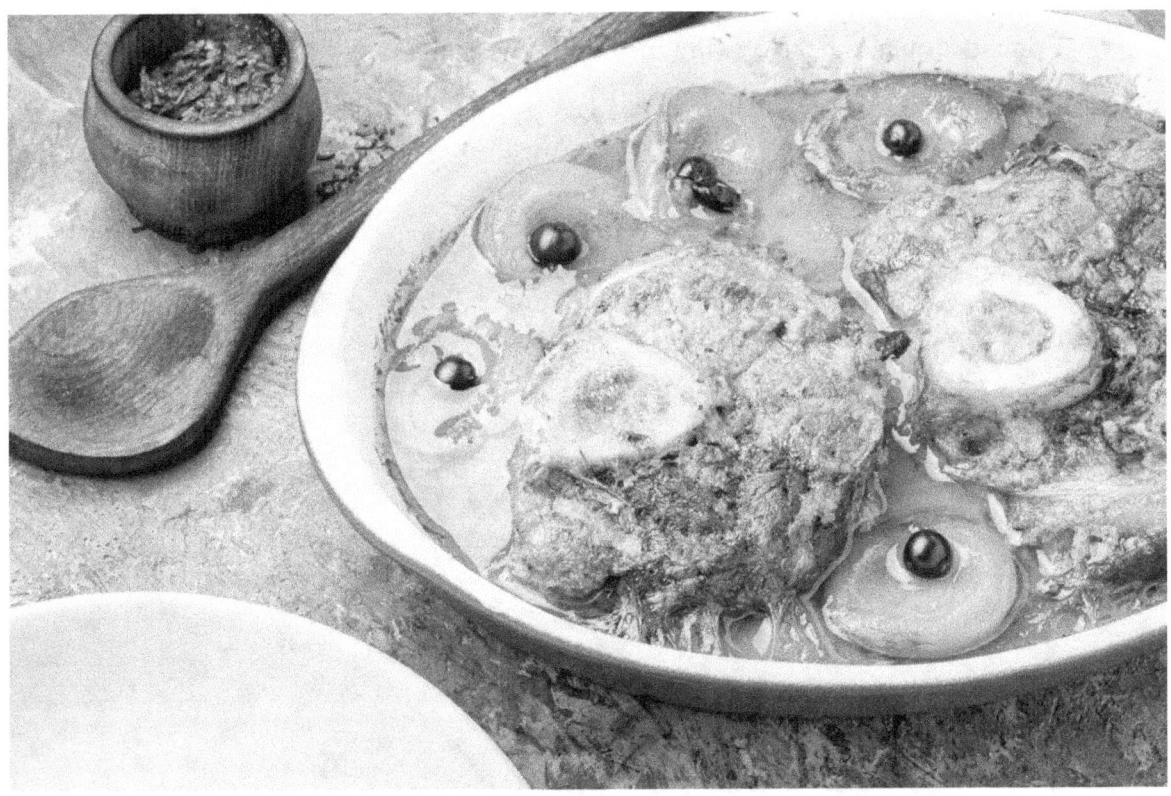

Celebrate reaching the final phase of stabilization and prepare this delicious beef stew for family and friends.

Servings: 6

Total Time: 1hour 15mins

Ingredients:

- 2 tbsp canola oil
- 1 pound 8 ounces beef stewing meat (cut into cubes)
- 1 medium onion (peeled and sliced)
- 3 cloves garlic (peeled and smashed)
- 1 cinnamon stick
- ½ tsp saffron
- 1 tbsp flour
- ¼ cups low-sodium beef stock
- 1 ½ cup dried apricots*
- Salt and black pepper
- 1½ tsp Tabasco

Directions:

Heat the oil in a frying pan.

Add the beef to the pan and sauté until browned all over.

Add the onion and garlic and sauté for 3-4 minutes, until browned.

Next, add the cinnamon stick and saffron, and cook for an additional 2 minutes.

Stir in the flour to combine.

Pour in the beef stock and apricots and simmer until the lamb is tender for approximately 60 minutes.

Remove and discard the cinnamon stick. Season to taste with salt and black pepper. Add a splash of Tabasco and enjoy.

*Soak the dried apricots in warm water until plumped up. Chop into pieces and use as directed.

Cook's Note: Consult with your surgeon or dietician to make sure this recipe is suitable for your pre or post-bariatric surgery diet plan and or phase.

Black Bean Corn Burgers

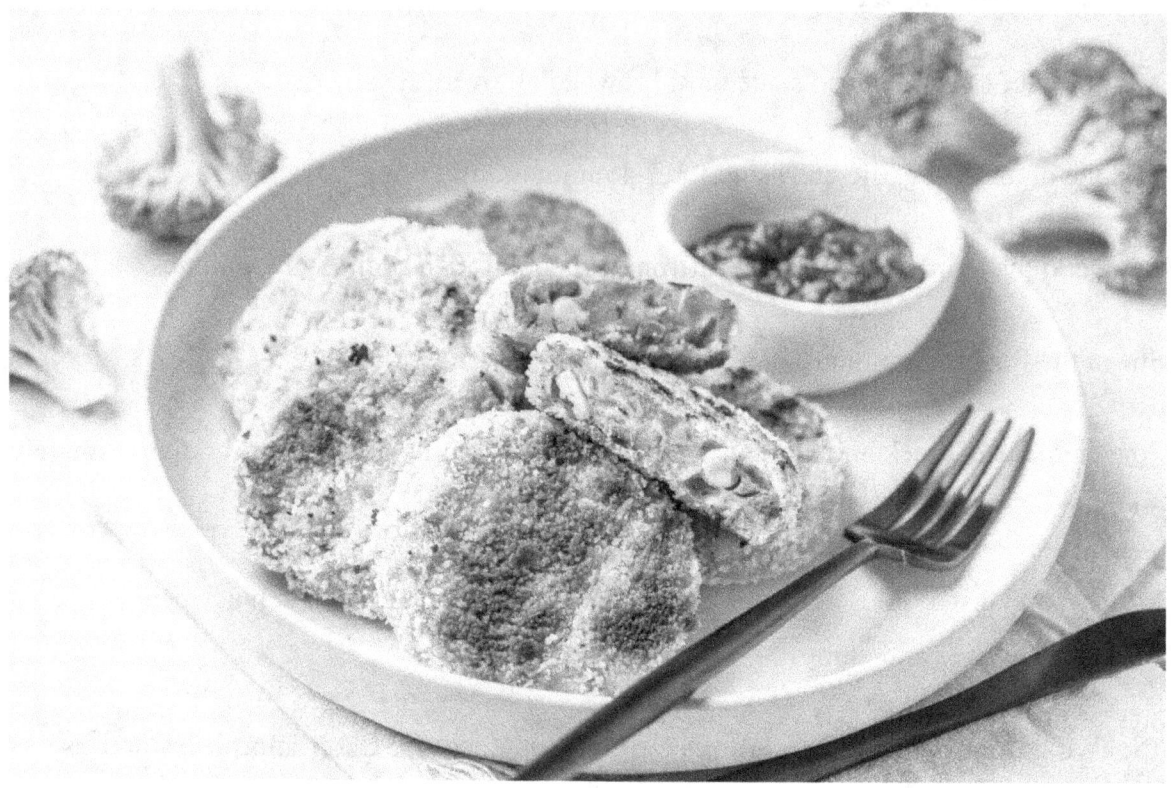

These meat-free burgers are cooked in healthy coconut oil spray and pan-fried to golden perfection.

Servings: 6

Total Time: 20mins

Ingredients:

- 1 small onion (peeled and chopped)
- 1 cup fresh or frozen corn kernels
- Nonstick coconut oil cooking spray
- 1 (14-ounce) can black beans (drained and rinsed)
- ⅓ cup tomato sauce
- 1 cup brown rice (cooked)
- 2 tsp ground cumin
- 1 tsp paprika
- 1 tsp chili powder
- 1 tsp salt (optional)
- Red pepper flakes (to season)
- ¼ cup rolled oats

Directions:

Add the onion and corn to a frying pan, and in nonstick coconut oil spray, sauté until soften and golden, for 10 minutes.

Add the black beans and tomato sauce to the pan, stir to combine, and warm through.

Add the brown rice to a food processor.

To the processor, add the black bean, onion, tomato paste, and corn mixture.

Add the cumin, paprika, chili powder, salt, and red pepper flakes, followed by the rolled oats and a splash of water. Pulse the mixture until thick, sticky, and textured. You may need to add 1-2 more tablespoons of rolled oats, if necessary, to achieve the desired consistency.

Shape the mixture into 6 patties, and pan-fry using nonstick coconut oil spray until browned on both sides.

Serve and enjoy.

Cook's Note: Consult with your surgeon or dietician to make sure this recipe is suitable for your pre or post-bariatric surgery diet plan and or phase.

Cauliflower Crust Turkey and Veg Pizza

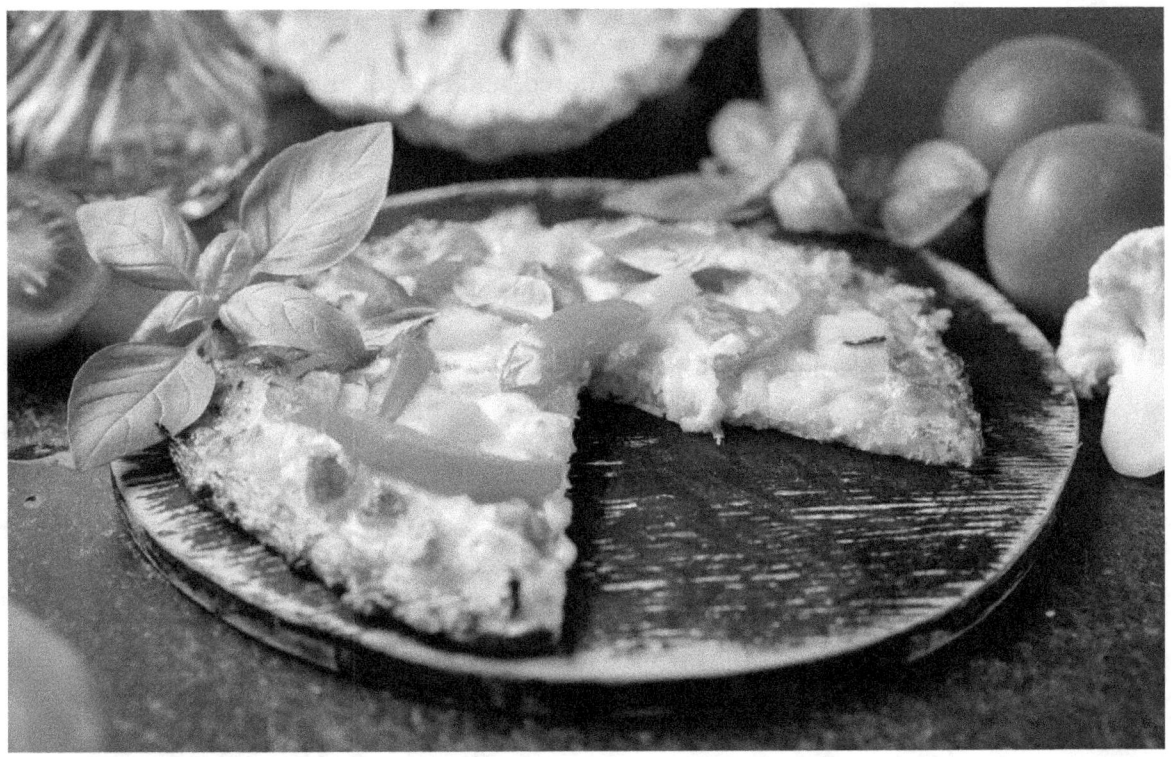

Once you have tasted this cauliflower crust pizza base, there is no going back to the regular kind. It's a real game changer!

Servings: 4

Total Time: 40mins

Ingredients:

Crust:

- 1 head cauliflower (leaves removed, cored, and coarsely chopped)
- 1 tsp Italian seasoning
- 1 tsp oregano
- Salt and black pepper
- 1 egg (beaten)
- 2 cloves garlic (peeled and minced)
- 1 cup 2% mozzarella cheese (shredded)

Toppings:

- 8 ounces 93% lean ground turkey
- ½ cup store-bought marinara sauce
- 1 small yellow squash (sliced)
- ½ cup mushrooms (sliced)
- ½ white onion (peeled and sliced)
- ½ cup 2% mozzarella (shredded)

Directions:

Preheat the main oven to 400 degrees F. Using aluminum foil, line a baking sheet.

Add the chopped cauliflower to a blender and on a high-speed process to a paste-like consistency. Transfer the mixture to a microwave-safe bowl and cook for approximately 5-6 minutes in the microwave.

In the meantime, in a pan, brown the turkey. Season the meat with Italian seasoning, oregano, salt, and black pepper.

When the cauliflower is cooked, add the remaining crust ingredients to the bowl (egg, garlic, and cheese). Mix well to combine and form a dough ball.

Using the back of a wooden spoon, spread the dough evenly onto the prepared baking sheet.

Bake the 'pizza' in the oven for 25 minutes. Remove from the oven and set the oven to broil.

Top the crust with marinara sauce, turkey, squash, mushrooms, and onion. Scatter the mozzarella over the top and place under the broiler for 4-6 minutes.

Take out of the oven and allow to cool slightly before serving.

Cook's Note: Consult with your surgeon or dietician to make sure this recipe is suitable for your pre or post-bariatric surgery diet plan and or phase.

Chicken Muffins

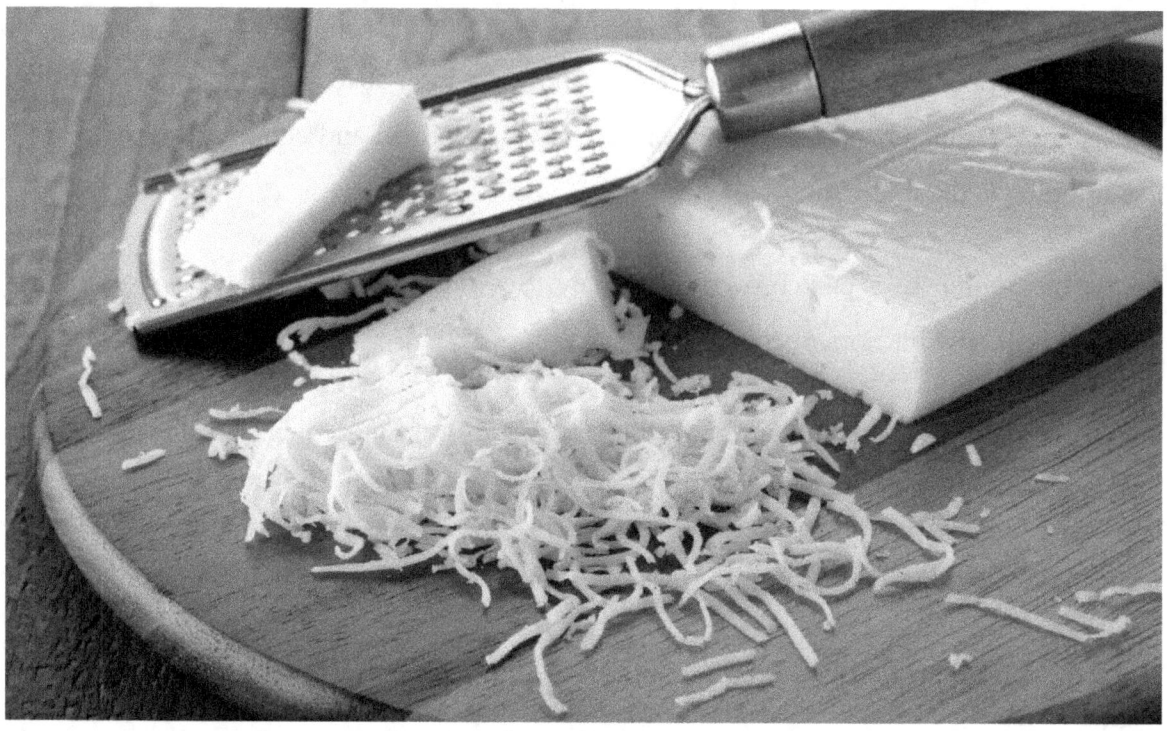

It's a good idea to plan working lunches ahead of time, and these chicken muffins are ideal for anyone with a busy workload. Pop one in your lunchbox and you are good to go.

Servings: 6

Total Time: 35mins

Ingredients:

- Nonstick baking spray
- 1 (12-ounce) can chicken (drained and flaked)
- 2 eggs
- ¼ cup celery (minced)
- 1 tsp dried minced onion
- ¼ tsp black pepper
- ½ tsp chicken seasoning
- 2 tbsp pimiento (mince)
- 2 ounces Cheddar cheese (shredded)

Directions:

Using a nonstick baking spray, grease a 6-cup muffin pan.

In a bowl, combine the canned chicken with the eggs, celery, dried minced onion, chicken seasoning, pimiento, and cheese.

Spoon the mixture into the prepared muffin pan.

Bake the muffins in the oven at 350 degrees F, until browned lightly, for 30-35 minutes.

Cook's Note: Consult with your surgeon or dietician to make sure this recipe is suitable for your pre or post-bariatric surgery diet plan and or phase.

Family-Friendly Meatloaf

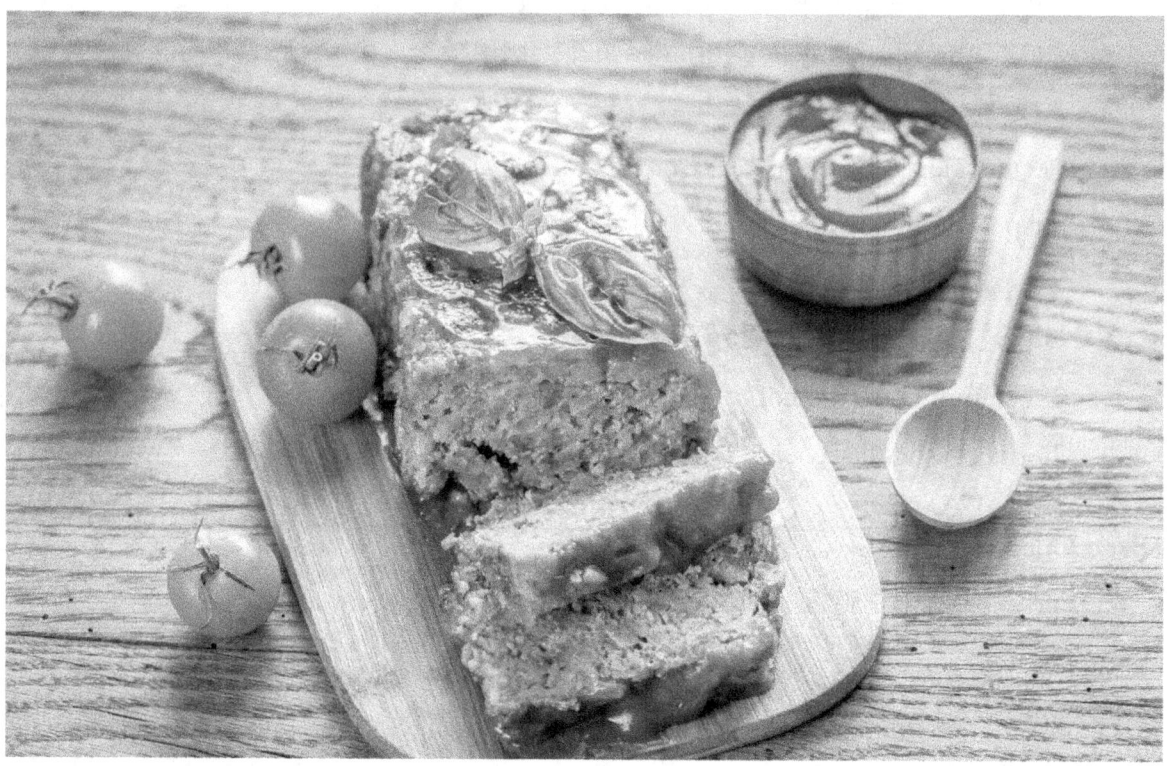

The key to successful weight loss does not have to prepare separate meals for the whole family, and this meatloaf recipe is suitable for everyone!

Servings: 8

Total Time: 1hour 20mins

Ingredients:

- 2 pounds lean ground beef
- 2 eggs
- ¼ cup reduced-carb ketchup
- 1 ½ tsp dry onion flakes
- 2 tsp salt
- ¼ tsp black pepper
- 4 ounces Cheddar cheese (shredded)

Glaze:

- ½ cup reduced-carb ketchup
- ¼ tsp dry mustard
- 2 tbsp granulated sugar-free sweetener

Directions:

In a bowl, combine the ground beef, eggs, ¼ cup ketchup, dry onion flakes, salt, black pepper, and Cheddar cheese.

Using aluminum foil, line a 9x5" loaf pan.

Press the meat mixture gently into the prepared pan, pushing the sides of the foil up to create a collar.

In a small bowl, combine the glaze ingredients (ketchup, dry mustard, and sweetener). Brush the glaze over the meatloaf in the pan.

Bake the meatloaf at 425 degrees F for 15 minutes.

Turn the oven temperature down to 325 degrees F, and bake for an additional 50 minutes until the meat registers an internal temperature of 145 degrees F.

Allow the meatloaf to rest for 3-4 minutes before serving.

Cook's Note: Consult with your surgeon or dietician to make sure this recipe is suitable for your pre or post-bariatric surgery diet plan and or phase.

Halibut in Parchment Paper

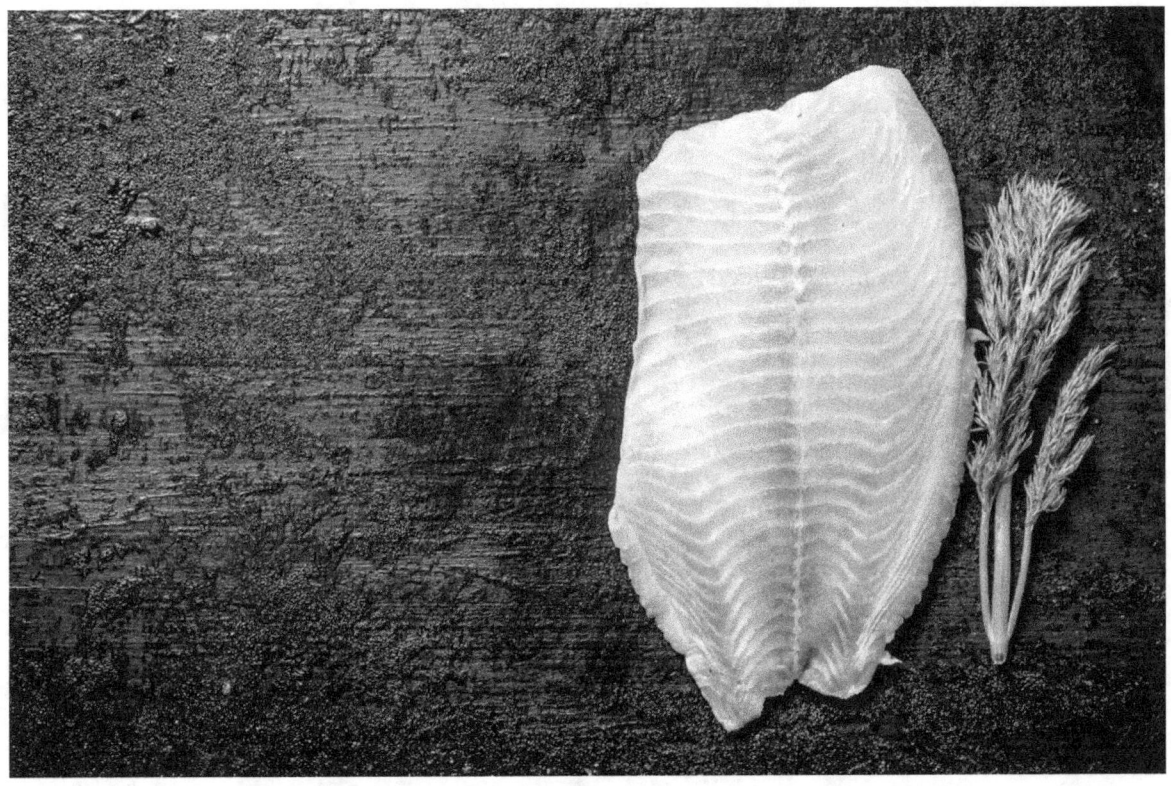

Cooking fish in parchment paper or, as they say in France, 'En Papilotte' seals in the flavor and natural juices. It also means a minimum amount of fat is needed for the baking process.

Servings: 2

Total Time: 20mins

Ingredients:

- 2 (4-ounce) halibut fillets
- 1 medium shallot (sliced into rings)
- 1 tsp garlic (peeled and minced)
- 1 tbsp canola oil
- 2 tsp capers
- ¼ cup fresh tomatoes (diced)
- 2 fresh tarragon sprigs
- ½ cup carrots (julienned)
- ½ cup red bell peppers (seeded and cut into fine strips)
- ½ cup celery (cut into fine strips)
- ½ cup leeks (cut into fine strips)
- ½ cup yellow squash (cut into fine strips)
- ¼ cup reduced-salt vegetable stock

Directions:

Preheat the main oven to 450 degrees F.

For each portion of fish, cut out a large circle of parchment paper. Fold the circles in half, and lay the fish on the seam. Top each portion with an equal amount of shallot, garlic, oil, capers, tomatoes, tarragon, carrots, red bell peppers, celery, leeks, and yellow squash.

Pour approximately 2 tablespoons of stock over each portion and fold the paper over, crimping to seal.

Lay each parchment parcel on a baking pan and bake in the preheated oven for 12-14 minutes, until the fish flakes easily when using a fork.

Serve and enjoy.

Cook's Note: Consult with your surgeon or dietician to make sure this recipe is suitable for your pre or post-bariatric surgery diet plan and or phase.

Middle Eastern Lamb

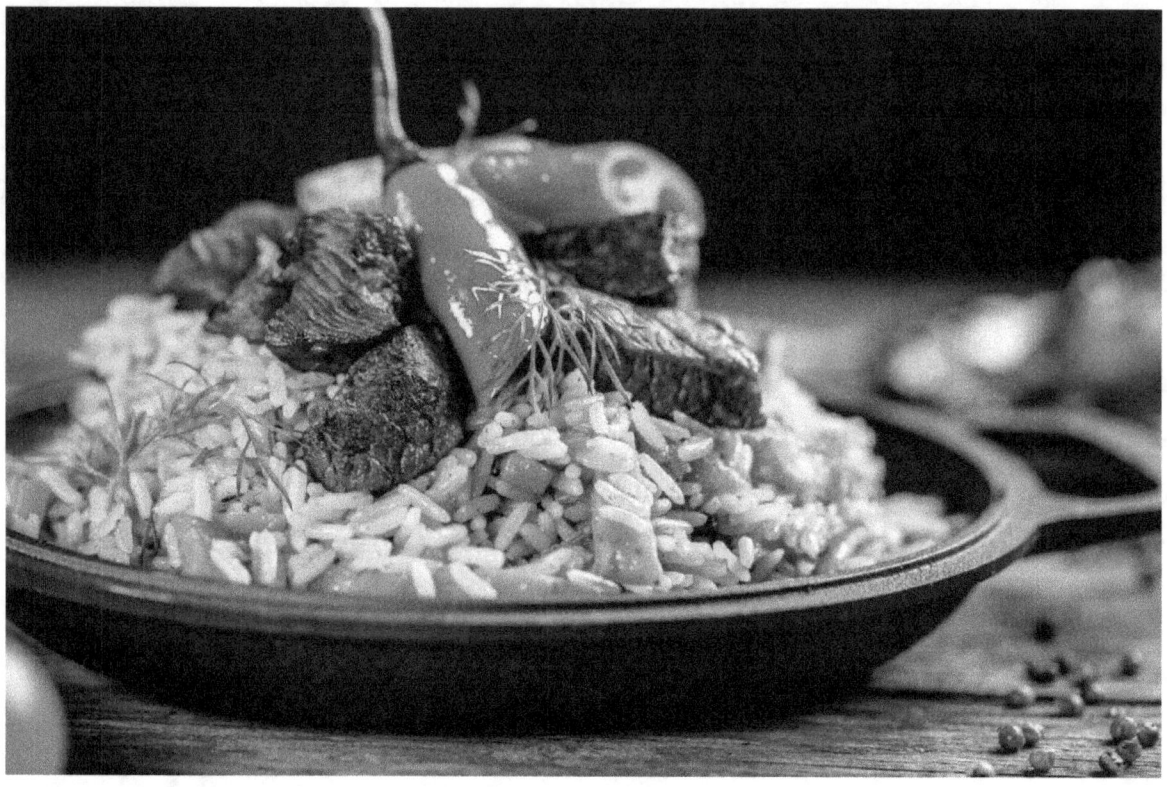

As long as it is trimmed of fat, chopped small, and chewed slowly, meat is still very much on the menu for weight loss patients during the stabilizing phase.

Servings: 4

Total Time: 45mins

Ingredients:

- 2 tsp olive oil
- 1 onion (peeled and sliced)
- 1 tsp ground cumin
- 1 tsp ground cinnamon
- 1 pound 2 ounces lamb (fat trimmed and diced)
- 1 potato (diced into cubes)
- 2 tbsp fresh mint (chopped)
- 1 tbsp lemon rind (finely grated)
- 1 cup reduced-salt beef stock
- 1 (14-ounce) no-salt-added canned and chopped tomatoes
- 1 tbsp runny honey
- 1 cup chickpeas (cooked)

Directions:

In a deep-sided frying pan or wok, over moderate heat, heat the oil.

To the pan, add the onion, ground cumin, and ground cinnamon. Stir-fry until the onions are softened for 3 minutes.

Add the lamb to the pan and stir-fry until browned, for 5 minutes.

Next, add the potatoes, fresh mint, lemon rind, beef stock, tomatoes, and honey.

Turn the heat down, cover with a lid and simmer for 15 minutes. Stir in the chickpeas and continue simmering for another 15 minutes or until the meat and potato are both tender.

Serve and enjoy.

Cook's Note: Consult with your surgeon or dietician to make sure this recipe is suitable for your pre or post-bariatric surgery diet plan and or phase.

Shrimp and Raspberry Salad

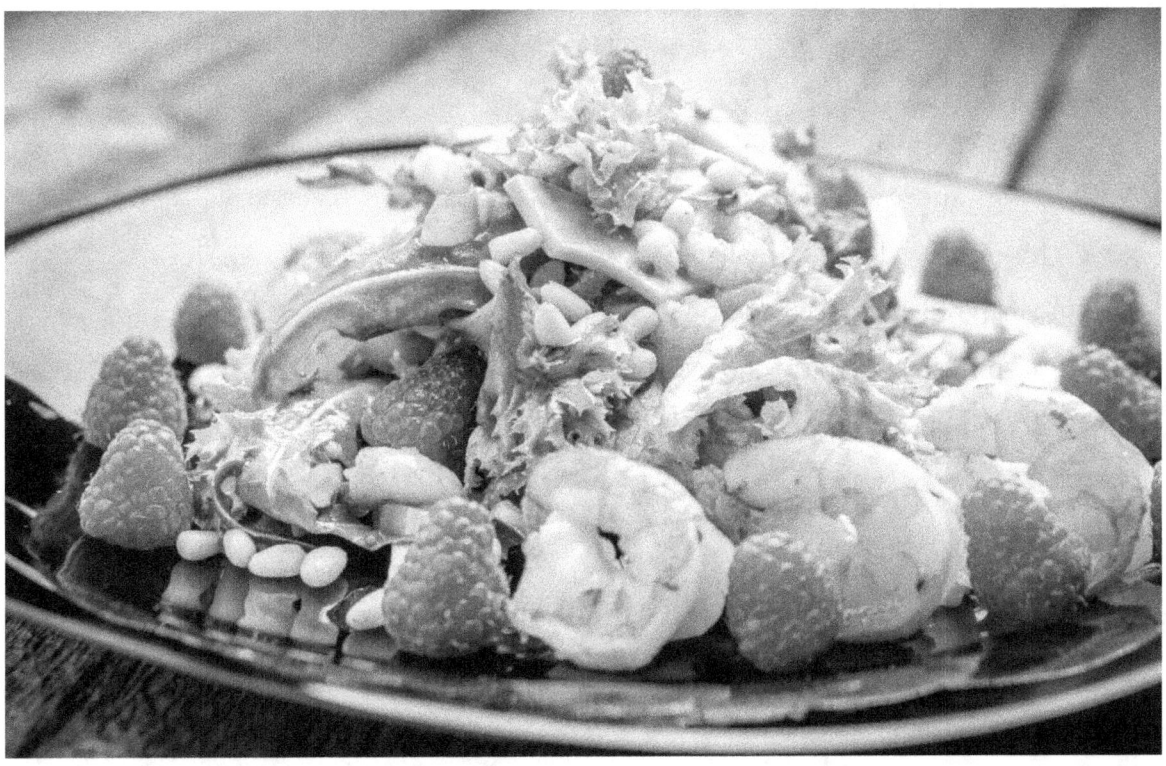

This seafood salad is as appealing to the eye as it is to the taste buds. Portion sizes for the future will be small, so every mouthful needs to count.

Servings: 1-2

Total Time: 1hour 10mins

Ingredients:

Marinade:

- 2 tsp sesame oil
- 1 clove garlic (peeled and finely chopped)
- Freshly squeezed juice and grated zest of 1 lime
- 1 tbsp reduced-salt soy sauce
- 1 small red chili (seed and finely chopped)
- 2 tbsp fresh coriander (chopped)
- Salt and black pepper

Salad:

- 1⅓ cups shrimp (shelled)
- A large handful of spinach leaves
- 1 ounce alfalfa sprouts
- ½ cup fresh raspberries
- ½ small red onion (peeled and thinly sliced)
- ½ small ripe avocado (peeled, pitted, and sliced)

Directions:

For the marinade: In a bowl, combine the sesame oil with garlic, fresh lime juice, lime zest, soy sauce, red chili, and coriander. Season the mixture to taste with salt and black pepper.

Remove approximately ¼ of the mixture and set it aside to use as a dressing.

Add the shrimp to the remaining mixture and transfer to the fridge for 60 minutes to marinade.

Thread the prawns onto metal skewers and broil lightly for 2-3 seconds on each side. Drizzle with around half of the marinade, set aside for dressing, in Step 2.

Add the spinach leaves and alfalfa to a bowl, and toss with any remaining set aside marinade.

Add the shrimp to the greens, followed by the raspberries, red onion, and avocado. Gently toss to combine, and enjoy.

Cook's Note: Consult with your surgeon or dietician to make sure this recipe is suitable for your pre or post-bariatric surgery diet plan and or phase.

Taco Casserole

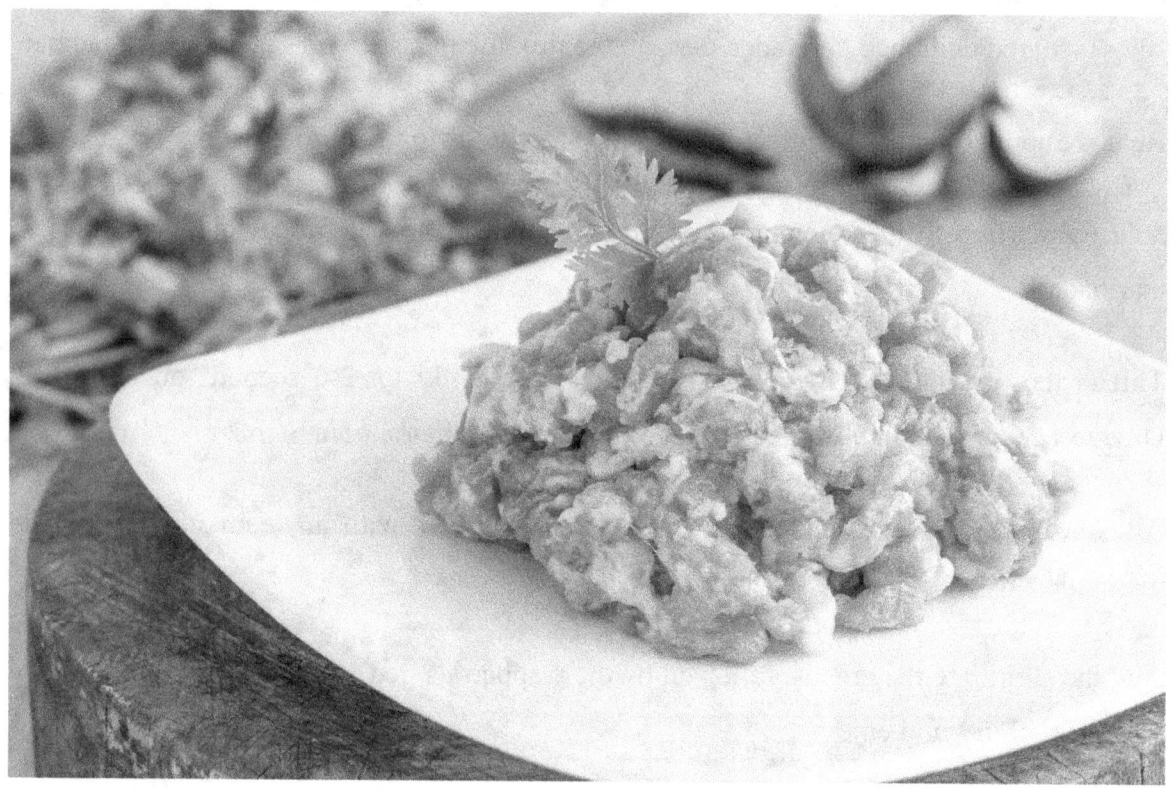

This tasty taco casserole is bariatric surgery-friendly and even better; you can share it with the whole family.

Servings: 8-10

Total Time: 1hour

Ingredients:

- Nonstick cooking spray
- 1 small zucchini (diced)
- 1 clove garlic (peeled and minced)
- 1 pound ground turkey
- 10 ounces canned black beans (drained and rinsed)
- 8 ounces canned tomatoes with chilies
- 1 (1-ounce) package reduced-sodium taco seasoning
- 8 ounces fat-free canned refried beans
- 2 cups Mexican blend cheese
- Reduced-fat sour cream (to serve, optional)

Directions:

Preheat the main oven to 350 degrees F.

Using nonstick cooking spray, spritz a frying pan.

Set the pan over moderate heat and when hot, add the zucchini and garlic and sauté until softened. Drain off any excess liquid and transfer the mixture to a bowl.

Add the turkey to the pan, and brown all over. Drain the meat and transfer to the bowl containing the zucchini and garlic. Stir in the black beans and canned tomatoes with chilies.

Fold in the taco seasoning to coat evenly, and transfer the mixture to a 13x9" baking dish.

Spread the refried beans in an even layer over the top.

Scatter the cheese over the beans and bake in the preheated oven for approximately 25-30 minutes or until the cheese melts and browns slightly.

Remove from the oven and allow to cool for several minutes before slicing.

Serve with a bowl of sour cream, and enjoy.

Cook's Note: Consult with your surgeon or dietician to make sure this recipe is suitable for your pre or post-bariatric surgery diet plan and or phase.

Author's Afterthoughts

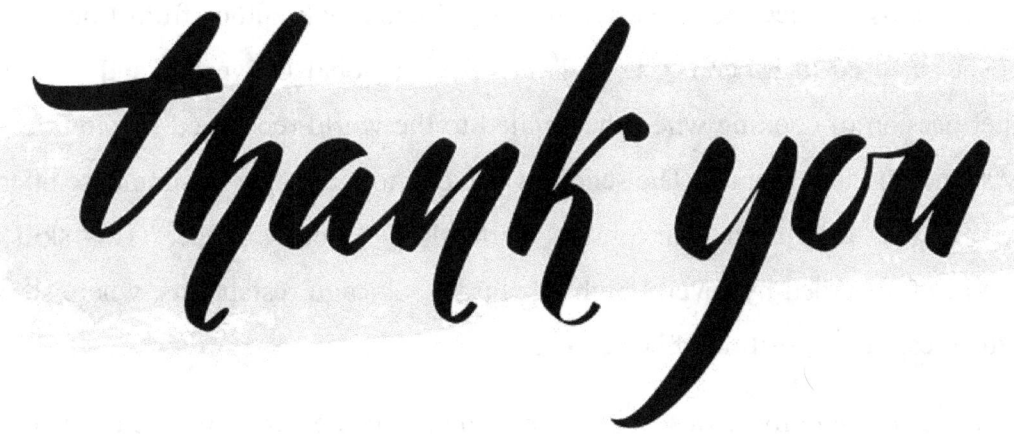

I would like to express my deepest thanks to you, the reader, for making this investment in one my books. I cherish the thought of bringing the love of cooking into your home.

With so much choice out there, I am grateful you decided to Purch this book and read it from beginning to end.

Please let me know by submitting an Amazon review if you enjoyed this book and found it contained valuable information to help you in your culinary endeavors. Please take a few minutes to express your opinion freely and honestly. This will help others make an informed decision on purchasing and provide me with valuable feedback.

Thank you for taking the time to review!

Christina Tosch

About the Author

Christina Tosch is a successful chef and renowned cookbook author from Long Grove, Illinois. She majored in Liberal Arts at Trinity International University and decided to pursue her passion of cooking when she applied to the world renowned Le Cordon Bleu culinary school in Paris, France. The school was lucky to recognize the immense talent of this chef and she excelled in her courses, particularly Haute Cuisine. This skill was recognized and rewarded by several highly regarded Chicago restaurants, where she was offered the prestigious position of head chef.

Christina and her family live in a spacious home in the Chicago area and she loves to grow her own vegetables and herbs in the garden she lovingly cultivates on her sprawling estate. Her and her husband have two beautiful children, 3 cats, 2 dogs and a parakeet they call Jasper. When Christina is not hard at work creating beautiful meals for Chicago's elite, she is hard at work writing engaging e-books of which she has sold over 1500.

Make sure to keep an eye out for her latest books that offer helpful tips, clear instructions and witty anecdotes that will bring a smile to your face as you read!

www.ingramcontent.com/pod-product-compliance
Lightning Source LLC
Chambersburg PA
CBHW080501220526
45465CB00006B/2344